American Academy of Orthopaedic Surgeons
6300 North River Road
Rosemont, Illinois 60018
1-800-626-6726

Arthroscopic Meniscal Repair

EDITED BY
W. DILWORTH CANNON, MD
Professor of Clinical Orthopaedic Surgery
Director of Sports Medicine
University of California, San Francisco
San Francisco, California

CONTRIBUTORS

Steven P. Arnoczky, DVM
W. Dilworth Cannon, MD
Scott A. Rodeo, MD
Thomas D. Rosenberg, MD

SERIES EDITOR
Thomas R. Johnson, MD

Director, Department of Publications
Marilyn L. Fox, PhD

Senior Editor
Joan Abern

Production Manager
Loraine Edwalds

Assistant Production Manager
Sophie Tosta

Production Assistant
Vanessa Villarreal

Graphic Design Coordinator
Pamela Hutton Erickson

The American Academy of Orthopaedic Surgeons Monograph Series is dedicated to Wendy O. Schmidt, American Academy of Orthopaedic Surgeons senior medical editor, 1987-1991.

ARTHROSCOPIC MENISCAL REPAIR
American Academy of Orthopaedic Surgeons®

The material presented in *Arthroscopic Meniscal Repair* has been made available by the American Academy of Orthopaedic Surgeons® for educational purposes only. This material is not intended to present the only, or necessarily best, methods or procedures for the medical situations discussed, but rather is intended to represent an approach, view, statement, or opinion of the author(s) or producer(s), which may be helpful to others who face similar situations.

Some drugs or medical devices demonstrated in Academy print or electronic publications have not been cleared by the Food and Drug Administration (FDA) or have been cleared by the FDA for specific uses only. The FDA has stated that it is the responsibility of the physician to determine the FDA clearance status of each drug or device he or she wishes to use in clinical practice.

Furthermore, any statements about commercial products are solely the opinion of the author(s) and do not represent an Academy endorsement or evaluation of these products. These statements may not be used in advertising or for any commercial purpose.

First Edition
Copyright © 1999 by the
American Academy of Orthopaedic Surgeons®

ISBN 0-89203-213-8

CONTENTS

PREFACE   vii

INTRODUCTION   1

BASIC SCIENCE CONSIDERATIONS   2

MENISCAL HEALING   7

TECHNIQUES OF MENISCUS REPAIR   12

SUMMARY   53

REFERENCES   53

INDEX   59

CONTRIBUTORS

Steven P. Arnoczky, DVM
Wade O. Brinker Endowed Professor of Surgery
Director, Laboratory for Comparative Orthopaedic Research
Professor of Orthopaedic Surgery, College of Human Medicine
Professor of Orthopaedic Surgery, College of Osteopathic Medicine
Michigan State University
East Lansing, Michigan

W. Dilworth Cannon, MD
Professor of Clinical Orthopaedic Surgery
Director of Sports Medicine
University of California, San Francisco
San Francisco, California

Scott A. Rodeo, MD
Assistant Attending Orthopaedic Surgeon
Assistant Scientist, Dept of Research
The Hospital For Special Surgery
New York, New York

Thomas D. Rosenberg, MD
The Orthopedic Specialty Hospital
Salt Lake City, Utah

PREFACE

Orthopaedic surgeons actively involved in the care of injuries of the knee, especially those associated with ligamentous tears, are faced with the problem of how to handle associated meniscus tears. It is often too easy to perform a partial meniscectomy because of possible time constraints in the operating room or economic factors, rather than to perform the much more complex arthroscopic meniscal repair. Charles E. Henning can be credited with performing the first arthroscopic meniscal repair in North America in February 1980. His technique is still an excellent one today, and although certain aspects of the method are difficult and time consuming, I believe his technique offers the surgeon the greatest degree of flexibility in handling the more complex reparable tears. During the 1980s and 90s, a number of alternative techniques have been developed, making arthroscopic meniscal repair easier and quicker. Today, the sports medicine surgeon should aggressively pursue meniscal repair whenever feasible in patients with associated ACL tears.

In this monograph, I have asked experts in their fields to contribute. Steven P. Arnoczky has written on the basic science of meniscal repair. I have followed with a detailed description of the Henning technique along with results of clinical studies. I also wrote the section following, with Thomas D. Rosenberg's help, on the zone-specific method of repair. Scott Rodeo then details the outside-in technique. I conclude with a section on the various all-inside methods currently available.

This monograph has extensive references, and is well illustrated in order to help the reader comprehend the subtleties of the various techniques of arthroscopic meniscal repair.

I want to acknowledge and thank the Academy staff for their encouragement and editing of this monograph. Special thanks should go to Joan Abern, Senior Editor, who edited the manuscript and managed the author review. Pamela Erickson, Graphic Design Coordinator, Loraine Edwalds, Production Manager, and Sophie Tosta, Assistant Production Manager also contributed their efforts in producing this attractive monograph.

W. DILWORTH CANNON, MD

ARTHROSCOPIC MENISCAL REPAIR

INTRODUCTION

This monograph will cover the history of meniscal repair; the basic science, including anatomy, blood supply, and function; meniscal healing; and the different types of arthroscopic meniscal repair, including inside-out, outside-in, and all-inside techniques. Results of these techniques will also be discussed.

Thomas Annandale,[1] in 1866, was the first person to perform an open meniscectomy. He followed this achievement by performing the first meniscus repair in 1883, when he sutured back the anterior horn of the medial meniscus in a miner. This surgery was considered successful when 10 weeks later, the patient returned to work with his knee apparently functioning normally. This feat went unappreciated. Bland-Sutton[2] believed that the menisci were only "functionless remains of leg muscle origins." In the early 1930s, Don King saw a patient with a unicompartmental gonarthrosis, and was told that the patient's meniscus had been excised in 1913. King went to the laboratory, found the patient's meniscus specimen in a bottle, and deduced that there was probably a relationship between the patient's arthritis and the absence of his meniscus. This reasoning prompted King's now famous studies on the canine meniscus, which culminated in his 2 publications in 1936, on the function and the healing of the meniscus.[3,4] King established that the amount of degenerative changes in the knee joint after meniscectomy was related to the amount of meniscus removed. He also found that meniscal tears healed in the avascular portion of the menisci if the tears extended into the well-vascularized meniscosynovial junction (Fig. 1). Years later surgeons began to honor his work. This recognition resulted in more partial meniscectomies than total meniscectomies being performed, and eventually in the repair of menisci. In 1948, Fairbank[5] showed that after meniscectomy, radiographic changes of joint space narrowing, ridging, and flattening occurred.

Subsequently, there were a plethora of reports documenting the premature development of arthritis after total meniscectomy, and to a lesser extent, after partial meniscectomy.[6–20] Cox,[13] in a canine study, showed that the development of arthritis was proportional to the amount of meniscus tissue removed. Lynch and associates[16] and Sommerlath[20] showed that meniscal repair resulted in a significantly lower incidence of arthritis compared to partial or total meniscectomy. In a recent study, Burks and associates[21] showed 88%

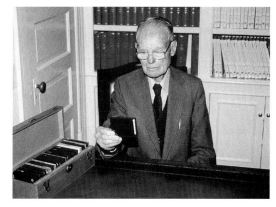

FIGURE 1
The late Don King, MD, studying his slides depicting the canine meniscus sections from his work in the early 1930s. (Courtesy of WD Cannon, MD)

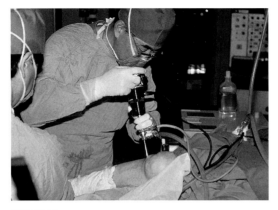

FIGURE 2
Hiroshi Ikeuchi, MD, performing arthroscopic surgery at the Tokyo Teishin Hospital where he had performed the first arthroscopic meniscus repair. (Courtesy of WD Cannon, MD)

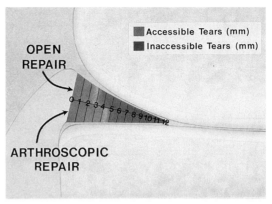

FIGURE 3
Arthroscopic versus open repair. The upper half of the meniscus shows the accessibility of the meniscus to open repair. The surgeon cannot gain access to tears that have rim widths greater than 2.5 to 3.0 mm. In contrast, arthroscopic techniques can repair meniscal tears with rim widths greater than 4.0 mm. Drawing courtesy of Jeanne Koelling. (Reproduced with permission from Cannon WD: Arthroscopic meniscal repair, in McGinty JB (ed): *Operative Arthroscopy*. New York, NY, Lippincott-Raven Press, 1991, p 237.)

good and excellent results in a group of 111 anterior cruciate ligament (ACL)-intact patients who had undergone partial meniscectomy an average of 14.7 years earlier. This finding was in sharp contrast to the 48% good and excellent results after partial meniscectomy in ACL-deficient patients.

In 1969, Hiroshi Ikeuchi[22] performed the first arthroscopic meniscal repair in Tokyo (Fig. 2). In the 1970s, DeHaven[23] and others[24–27] began to do open meniscal repair through a posterior incision. One disadvantage to the open technique is that it limits access to the mobile meniscal fragment, limiting this type of repair to rim widths no greater than 2.5 to 3.0 mm (Fig. 3). After Henning[28] performed the first arthroscopic meniscal repair in North America in 1980, surgeons began to take notice of this technique (Fig. 4). No longer was meniscus repair limited to small rim widths in the posterior horn, but now a wide variety of meniscus tears could be repaired that previously were excised. Henning's original technique[28] was, and still is, difficult in the hands of most surgeons. In a short period of time, other techniques making meniscus repair more easily accomplished were introduced.[29–37] Sommerlath,[20] analyzing matched pairs of 50 patients in a follow-up of 6 to 9 years, found that the group that had had open meniscal repair had significantly less arthritis than the group that had undergone partial meniscectomy.

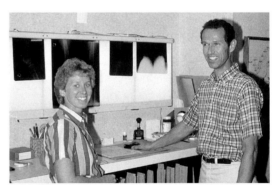

FIGURE 4
The late Charles E. Henning, MD, at his office in Wichita, Kansas. Dr. Henning performed the first arthroscopic meniscal repair in North America in 1980. (Courtesy of WD Cannon, MD)

BASIC SCIENCE CONSIDERATIONS

The menisci are C-shaped disks of fibrocartilage interposed between the condyles of the femur and tibia. Once described as the functionless remains of leg muscle[2] the menisci are now realized to be integral components in the complex biomechanics of the knee joint.[38] This realization has resulted in a renewed interest in the basic science of the meniscus in terms of its structure, function, and physiology. This section will examine some of these basic science aspects of the human meniscus.

GROSS ANATOMY

The menisci of the knee joint are actually extensions of the tibia that serve to deepen the articular surfaces of the tibial plateau to better accommodate the condyles of the femur. The peripheral border of each meniscus is thick, convex, and attached to the capsule of the joint; the inside border tapers to a thin free edge[39] (Fig. 5). The proximal surfaces of the menisci are concave and in contact with the condyles of the femur; their distal surfaces are flat and rest on the tibia.

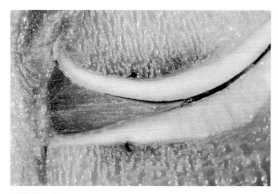

FIGURE 5
Frontal section of the medial compartment of a human knee illustrating the articulation of the menisci with the condyles of the femur and tibia. (Reproduced with permission from Warren RF, Arnoczky SP, Wickiewicz TL: Anatomy of the knee, in Nicholas JA, Hershman EB (eds): *The Lower Extremity and Spine in Sports Medicine.* St. Louis, MO, CV Mosby, 1986, pp 657–694.)

The medial meniscus is somewhat semicircular in form. It is approximately 3.5 cm in length and considerably wider posteriorly than it is anteriorly[39] (Fig. 6). The anterior horn of the medial meniscus is attached to the tibial plateau in the area of the anterior intercondylar fossa in front of the ACL. The posterior fibers of the anterior horn attachment merge with the transverse ligament, which connects the anterior horns of the medial and lateral menisci. The posterior horn of the medial meniscus is firmly attached to

the posterior intercondylar fossa of the tibia between the attachments of the lateral meniscus and the posterior cruciate ligament. The periphery of the medial meniscus is attached to the joint capsule throughout its length. The tibial portion of the capsular attachment is often referred to as the coronary ligament. At its midpoint, the medial meniscus is more firmly attached to the femur and tibia through a condensation in the joint capsule known as the deep medial collateral ligament.

The lateral meniscus is almost circular and covers a larger portion of the tibial articular surface than the medial meniscus; it is approximately the same width from front to back. The anterior horn of the lateral meniscus is attached to the tibia in front of the intercondylar eminence and behind the attachment of the ACL, with which it partially blends. The posterior horn of the lateral meniscus is attached behind the intercondylar eminence of the tibia in front of the posterior end of the medial meniscus. Although there is no attachment of the lateral meniscus to the lateral collateral ligament, there is a loose peripheral attachment to the joint capsule.[39]

Several ligaments run from the posterior horn of the lateral meniscus to the medial femoral condyle, either just in front of or behind the origin of the posterior cruciate ligament. These are

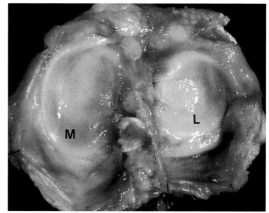

FIGURE 6
Photograph of a tibial plateau showing the shape and attachments of the medial (M) and lateral (L) menisci. (Reproduced with permission from Warren RF, Arnoczky SP, Wickiewicz TL: Anatomy of the knee, in Nicholas JA, Hershman EB (eds): *The Lower Extremity and Spine in Sports Medicine.* St Louis, MO, CV Mosby, 1986, pp 657–694.)

known as the anterior meniscofemoral ligament (ligament of Humphrey) and the posterior meniscofemoral ligament (ligament of Wrisberg).

ULTRASTRUCTURE AND BIOCHEMISTRY

Histologically, the meniscus is a fibrocartilaginous tissue composed, primarily, of an interlacing network of collagen fibers interposed with cells. In addition, the extracellular matrix consists of proteoglycan molecules and glycoproteins.

The cells of the meniscus are responsible for synthesizing and maintaining the extracellular matrix. There is still some debate as to whether the cells of the meniscus are fibroblasts, chondrocytes, or a mixture of both and whether the tissue should be classified as fibrous tissue or fibrocartilage.[40] The cells have been termed fibrochondrocytes because of their chondrocytic appearance and their ability to synthesize a fibrocartilage matrix. Two basic types of fibrochondrocytes within the meniscus have been described: a fusiform cell found in the superficial zone of the meniscus and an ovoid, or polygonal, cell found throughout the remainder of the tissue.[41] Although the fusiform cells resemble fibroblasts, they are situated in well-formed lacunae and resemble the chondrocytes found in the superficial (tangential) zone of articular cartilage.[40,41] Both cell types contain abundant endoplasmic reticulum and Golgi complexes. Mitochondria are only occasionally visualized, suggesting that, as in articular chondrocytes, the major pathway for energy production for the fibrochondrocytes in their avascular surroundings is probably anaerobic glycolysis.[42]

The extracellular matrix of the meniscus is composed primarily of collagen (60% to 70% of the dry weight).[43] It is mainly type I collagen (90%), although types II, III, V, and VI have been identified within the meniscus.[43] The circumferential orientation of these collagen fibers appears to be directly related to the function of the meniscus. In a classic study describing the orientation of the collagen fibers within the menisci, it was noted that although the principal orientation of the collagen fibers is circumferential, a few small, radially disposed fibers appear on both the femoral and tibial surfaces of the menisci as well as within the substance of the tissue.[44] It is theorized that these radial fibers act as "ties" to provide structural rigidity and help resist longitudinal splitting of the menisci resulting from undue compression. Subsequent light and electron microscopic examinations of the menisci revealed 3 different collagen framework layers: a superficial layer composed of a network of fine fibrils woven into a mesh-like matrix, a surface layer just beneath the superficial layer composed, in part, of irregularly aligned collagen bundles, and a middle layer in which the collagen fibers are larger and coarser and are oriented in a parallel, circumferential direction[45,46] (Fig. 7). It is this middle layer that allows the meniscus to resist tensile forces and function as a transmitter of load across the knee joint.

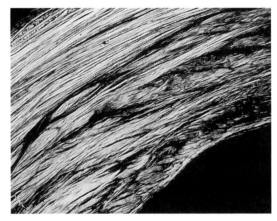

FIGURE 7
Photomicrograph of a longitudinal section of a human medial meniscus illustrating the predominantly circumferential orientation of the collagen fibers (hematoxylin & eosin × 40 under polarized light). (Reproduced with permission from Woo SL-Y, An KN, Arnoczky SP, Wayne JS, Fithian DC, Myers BS: Anatomy, biology, and biomechanics of tendon, ligament, and meniscus, in Simon SR (ed): *Orthopaedic Basic Science*. Rosemont, IL, 1994, American Academy of Orthopaedic Surgeons, pp 45-87.)

In addition to collagen, the extracellular matrix of the meniscus also consists of proteoglycans, matrix glycoproteins, and elastin.[47,48] The proteoglycan content of the adult meniscus is approximately 10% of that in hyaline cartilage, although this has been shown to vary with age and location within the tissue. A study in the porcine meniscus has shown a higher (2 to 4 times) content of hexosamine and uronic acid in the inner third of the meniscus as compared to the outer two thirds.[49] There was also a trend toward higher concentrations in the anterior horn as compared to the posterior horn in both the medial and lateral menisci.[49] The glycosaminoglycan profile of the adult human meniscus has been reported to be: chondroitin 6-sulfate (40%), chondroitin 4-sulfate (10% to 20%), dermatan sulfate (20% to 30%), and keratan sulfate (15%).[50–52]

Matrix glycoproteins, such as the link proteins, which stabilize the proteoglycan-hyaluronic acid aggregates and a 116-kd protein of unknown consequence, have also been identified within the extracellular matrix.[53] In addition, adhesive glycoproteins such as type VI collagen,[42] fibronectin,[42] and thrombospondin,[54] have also been isolated from the meniscus. These macromolecules have the property to bind to other matrix macromolecules and/or cell surfaces and may play a role in the supramolecular organization of the extracellular molecules of the meniscus.[42]

MENISCAL FUNCTION

The meniscus has been shown to play a vital role in load transmission across the knee joint. Biomechanical studies have demonstrated that at least 50% of the compressive load of the knee joint is transmitted through the meniscus in extension, whereas approximately 85% of the load is transmitted in 90° of flexion.[55] In the meniscectomized knee, the contact area is reduced approximately 50%.[55] This significantly increases the load per unit area and results in articular cartilage damage and degeneration. This evidence explains the osteophyte formation, joint space narrowing, and flattening of the femoral condyle that have been observed following total meniscectomy[5] (Fig. 8).

Partial meniscectomy has also been shown to significantly increase contact pressures.[56] It has been shown that resection of as little as 15% to 34% of the meniscus increased contact pressures by more than 350%.[57] Thus, even a partial meniscectomy can affect the ability of the meniscus to function in load transmission across the knee.

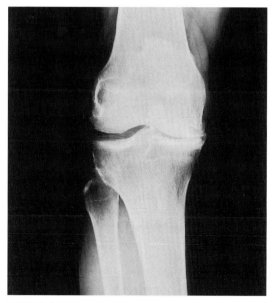

FIGURE 8
Radiograph illustrating collapse and degeneration of the medial compartment of the knee following total medial meniscectomy. (Reproduced with permission from Arnoczky SP, Cooper DE: Meniscal repair, in Goldberg VM (ed): *Controversies of Total Knee Arthroplasty.* New York, NY, Raven Press, 1991, pp 291–302.)

Another proposed function of the meniscus is that of shock absorption. It has been suggested that the viscoelastic menisci may function to dampen the load generated during walking.[57,58] Experimental studies have shown that the normal knee has a shock-absorbing capacity about 20% higher than that of knees that have undergone meniscectomy.[58] Because the inability of a joint system to absorb shock has been strongly implicated in the development of osteoarthritis,[59] the meniscus appears to play an important role in maintaining the health of the knee.

The menisci are also believed to contribute to knee joint stability. Although medial meniscectomy alone does not increase anterior-posterior joint translation significantly, it has been demonstrated that medial meniscectomy in association with ACL insufficiency significantly increases anterior translation of the tibia.[60] However, lateral meniscectomy, alone or in association with ACL insufficiency, has not been shown to increase knee joint laxity.[61]

Because the menisci serve to increase the congruity between the condyles of the femur and tibia, they contribute significantly to overall joint conformity. It has been suggested that this function assists in the overall lubrication of the articular surfaces of the knee joint.

Finally, the menisci may serve as proprioceptive structures providing a feedback mechanism for joint position sense. This has been inferred from the presence of type I and II nerve endings observed in the anterior and posterior horns of the meniscus.

VASCULAR ANATOMY OF THE MENISCUS

The menisci of the knee are relatively avascular structures; their limited peripheral blood supply originates predominantly from the lateral and medial genicular arteries (both inferior and superior).[62] Branches from these vessels give rise to a perimeniscal capillary plexus within the synovial and capsular tissues of the knee joint. This plexus is an arborizing network of vessels that supplies the peripheral border of the meniscus throughout its attachment to the joint capsule[62] (Fig. 9). These perimeniscal vessels are oriented in a predominantly circumferential pattern with radial branches directed toward the center of the joint (Fig. 10). Anatomic studies have shown that the degree of vascular penetration is 10% to 30% of the width of the medial meniscus and 10% to 25% of the width of the lateral meniscus.[62]

The middle genicular artery, along with a few terminal branches of the medial and lateral genicular arteries, also supplies vessels to the meniscus through the vascular synovial covering of the anterior and posterior horn attachments (Fig. 11). These synovial vessels penetrate the horn attachments and give rise to endoligamentous vessels that enter the meniscal horns for a short distance and end in terminal capillary loops. A small reflection of vascular synovial tissue is also present throughout the peripheral attachment of the medial and lateral menisci on both the femoral and tibial articular surfaces. An exception is the posterolateral portion of the lateral meniscus adjacent to the area of the popliteal tendon (Fig. 12). This "synovial fringe" extends for a short distance (1 to 3 mm) over the articular surfaces of the

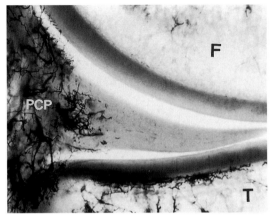

FIGURE 9

Five-millimeter thick frontal section of the medial compartment of the knee after vascular perfusion with India ink and tissue clearing with a modified Spalteholz technique. Branching radial vessels from the perimeniscal capillary plexus (PCP) can be seen penetrating the peripheral border of the medial meniscus. F = Femur, T = Tibia. (Reproduced with permission from Arnoczky SP, Warren RF: Microvasculature of the human meniscus. *Am J Sports Med* 1982;10:90–95.)

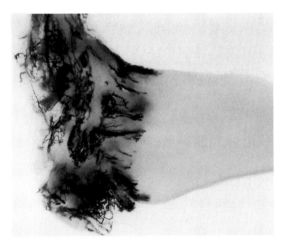

FIGURE 10

Three-millimeter thick transverse section of a medial meniscus (Spalteholz × 8) demonstrating the terminally looped capillary vessels and their penetration into the peripheral border of the meniscus. (Reproduced with permission from Arnoczky SP, Warren RF: Microvasculature of the human meniscus. *Am J Sports Med* 1982;10:90–95.)

menisci and contains small, terminally looped vessels. Although this vascular synovial tissue adheres intimately to the articular surfaces of the menisci, it does not contribute vessels into the meniscal tissue.[62]

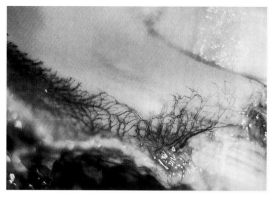

FIGURE 11
Anterior horn of an India ink-perfused medial meniscus showing the extension of the vascular synovial fringe into the synovial covering of the anterior horn attachment. (Reproduced with permission from Arnoczky SP, Warren RF: Microvasculature of the human meniscus. *Am J Sports Med* 1982;10:90–95.)

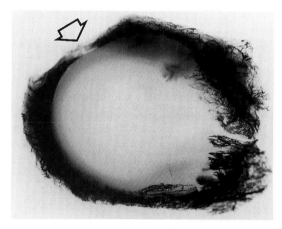

FIGURE 12
Superior aspect of the lateral meniscus following vascular perfusion with India ink and tissue clearing using a modified Spalteholz technique. Note the vascularity at the periphery of the menisci as well as at the anterior and posterior horn attachments. The absence of peripheral vasculature at the posterior corner of the lateral meniscus (arrow) represents the area of passage of the popliteal tendon. (Reproduced with permission from Arnoczky SP, Warren RF: Microvasculature of the human meniscus. *Am J Sports Med* 1982;10:90–95.)

MENISCAL HEALING

Thomas Annandale was credited with the first surgical repair of a torn meniscus in 1883,[1] but it was not until 1936, when King[3] published his classic experiment on meniscus healing in dogs, that the actual biologic limitations of meniscus healing were set forth. King demonstrated that, for meniscus lesions to heal, the lesion must communicate with the peripheral blood supply. Although the vascular supply of the meniscus is an essential element in determining its potential for repair; of equal importance is the ability of this blood supply to support the inflammatory response characteristic of wound repair. Clinical and experimental observations have demonstrated that the peripheral blood supply is capable of producing a reparative response similar to that observed in other connective tissues.[63]

After injury within the peripheral vascular zone, a fibrin clot forms that is rich in inflammatory cells. Vessels from the perimeniscal capillary plexus proliferate through this fibrin "scaffold," accompanied by the proliferation of undifferentiated mesenchymal cells. Eventually, the lesion is filled with a cellular, fibrovascular scar tissue that "glues" the wound edges together and appears continuous with the adjacent normal meniscal fibrocartilage (Fig. 13). Vessels from the perimeniscal capillary plexus, as well as the proliferative vascular pannus from the "synovial fringe," penetrate the fibrous scar to provide a marked inflammatory response (Fig. 14).

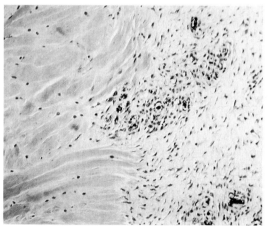

FIGURE 13
Photomicrograph of healing meniscus at the junction of the fibrovascular scar and the normal adjacent meniscal tissue (hematoxylin & eosin × 75). (Reproduced with permission from Arnoczky SP, Warren RF: The microvasculature of the meniscus and its response to injury: An experimental study in the dog. *Am J Sports Med* 1983;11:131–141.)

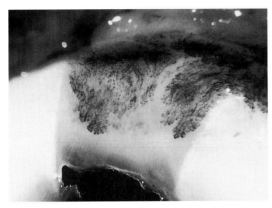

FIGURE 14

India ink-perfused canine medial meniscus showing the fibrovascular scar 6 weeks after complete radial transection. Notice the proliferation of vascular synovial tissue over the fibrovascular scar. (Reproduced with permission from Arnoczky SP, Warren RF: The microvasculature of the meniscus and its response to injury: An experimental study in the dog. *Am J Sports Med* 1983;11:131–141.)

Experimental studies have shown that radial lesions of the meniscus extending to the synovium are completely healed with fibrovascular scar tissue by 10 weeks[63] (Fig. 15). Modulation of this scar

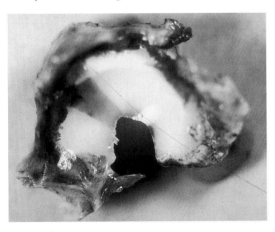

FIGURE 15

India ink-perfused canine medial meniscus 10 weeks following complete transection. The fibrovascular scar has completely filled the lesion and remodeled to the normal contours of the meniscus. Note that the response of the synovial fringe has subsided but injected vessels from the perimeniscal capillary plexus are still visible within the fibrovascular scar. (Reproduced with permission from Arnoczky SP, Warren RF: The microvasculature of the meniscus and its response to injury: An experimental study in the dog. *Am J Sports Med* 1983;11:131–141.)

into normal-appearing fibrocartilage, however, can require several months. It should be stressed that the initial strength of this repair tissue, as compared to the normal meniscus has been found to be minimal (33% at 8 weeks, 52% at 4 months, and 62% at 6 months).[64]

The ability of meniscal lesions to heal has provided the rationale for the repair of peripheral meniscal injuries, and numerous clinical reports have demonstrated excellent results after primary repair of peripheral meniscal injuries. Postoperative examinations of these peripheral repairs have revealed a process of repair similar to that noted in the experimental models.

When examining injured menisci for potential repair, lesions are often classified by the location of the tear relative to the blood supply of the meniscus and the "vascular appearance" of the peripheral and central surfaces of the tear. The so-called red-red tear (peripheral capsular detachment) has a functional blood supply on the capsular and meniscal side of the lesion and, obviously, has the best prognosis for healing. The red-white tear (meniscus rim tear through the peripheral vascular zone) has an active peripheral blood supply (Fig. 16), while the central (inner) surface of the lesion is devoid of functioning vessels. Theoretically, these lesions should have sufficient vascularity to heal by fibrovascular proliferation. The white-white tear (meniscus lesion completely in the avascular zone) has no blood supply and, theoretically, cannot heal.

Meniscus repair has generally been limited to the peripheral vascular area of the meniscus (red-red, red-white tears), but a significant number of lesions occur in the central, avascular portion of the meniscus (white-white tears). Experimental and clinical observations have shown that these lesions are incapable of healing and thus have provided the rationale for partial meniscectomy. In an effort to extend the level of repair into these avascular areas, techniques have been developed that provide vascularity to these white-white tears. These techniques include vascular access channels[63] and synovial abrasion.[65]

Initial attempts to extend the peripheral vascular response of the meniscus into the avascular

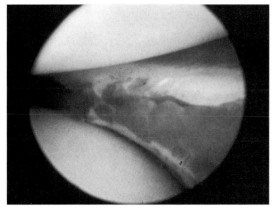

FIGURE 16

Arthroscopic view of a peripheral tear of a meniscus in the red-white zone. Note the vascular granulation tissue present at the margin of the lesion. (Courtesy R. Jackson) (Reproduced with permission from Arnoczky SP, Torzilli PA: The biology of cartilage, in Hunter LY, Fink RJ (eds): *Rehabilitation of the Injured Knee*. St. Louis, MO, CV Mosby, 1984, pp 148–252.)

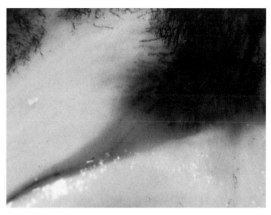

FIGURE 17

India ink-perfused canine medial meniscus 4 weeks after longitudinal incision and the creation of a vascular access channel. Vessels can be seen progressing within the fibrin clot in the anterior limb of the longitudinal lesion. (Reproduced with permission from: Arnoczky SP, Warren RF: The microvasculature of the meniscus and its response to injury: An experimental study in the dog. *Am J Sports Med* 1983;11:131–141.)

zone used the creation of vascular access channels.[63] This concept was based on the observation that when avascular lesions were extended into the peripheral blood supply of the meniscus, vessels would migrate into those lesions and heal them by fibrovascular proliferation.

In an experimental study in dogs, a longitudinal lesion in the avascular portion of the medial meniscus was connected, at its midportion, to the peripheral vasculature of the meniscus by a full-thickness vascular access channel.[63] Vessels from the peripheral tissues migrated into the channel and healed the meniscal lesion by the proliferation of fibrovascular scar tissue (Fig. 17). This same mechanism was successful in healing lesions in the avascular portion of rabbit menisci.[66] When using the vascular access technique it is imperative to remember that the function of the meniscus can be destroyed by cutting across the important circumferential collagen bundles making up the peripheral rim. However, because the vascularity extends into the meniscus at least 25% of its width, a vascular access channel can be created without completely disrupting the integrity of the peripheral rim of the meniscus.

Another means of manipulating the vascular supply of the meniscus that has found increasing clinical use is the technique of synovial abrasion. In this technique, the synovial fringe is abraded in an effort to incite a more robust vascular response near the site of the meniscal lesion.[65] As noted previously, the meniscal synovial fringe is a vascular synovial tissue that extends over the femoral and tibial articular surfaces of the meniscus. Although it does not contribute vessels to the meniscal stroma under normal circumstances, it plays a major role in the healing of meniscal lesions in contact with the peripheral vasculature of the meniscus. It has been theorized that by stimulating (through rasping or abrading) the synovial fringe, a proliferative vascular response could be extended over the meniscal surface to previously avascular areas of the meniscus (Fig. 18). Although clinical results have suggested an improved healing rate when synovial abrasion is used, the exact extent and character of the repair tissue has yet to be determined.

Finally, the use of an exogenous fibrin clot has been shown to heal avascular lesions without benefit of a blood supply in a canine model[38] (Fig. 19). Previous work had suggested that white-white tears in the meniscus were incapable of repair. This was based on the belief that the meniscal cells were incapable of mounting a repair response and

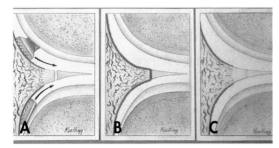

FIGURE 18
These drawings depict the healing response of rasping or abrading the perimeniscal synovium adjacent to a meniscus tear. Rasping of both the superior and inferior surfaces of the meniscosynovial junction **(A)** leads to a proliferation of synovium growing across the meniscus rim and into the tear site **(B).** Once healing has occurred, with further maturation, the synovium recedes **(C)**. (Drawings courtesy of Jeanne Koelling)

that a blood supply was a prerequisite for wound repair. However, in an experimental study, Webber and associates[67,68] demonstrated that meniscal fibrochondrocytes are capable of proliferation and matrix synthesis when exposed to chemotactic and mitogenic factors normally present in the wound hematoma. Using cell cultures, they demonstrated that meniscal cells exposed to platelet-derived growth factor were able to proliferate and synthesize an extracellular matrix.

In normal wound repair, hemorrhage from vascular injury gives rise to a fibrin clot that provides a scaffolding that supports a reparative response. In addition, the clot provides substances, such as platelet-derived growth factor and fibronectin, which act as chemotactic and mitogenic stimuli of reparative cells. Clinical use of the fibrin clot technique has suggested that it can improve the healing rate in meniscal tears.

Although the postoperative rehabilitation regimens following meniscal repair vary among surgeons, several basic science considerations must be taken into account when developing a postoperative protocol for meniscal repair.

MOTION

A classic study[69] has demonstrated that during knee flexion, the menisci translate posteriorly on the tibial plateau. The medial meniscus had a mean posterior translation of 5.1 mm and the lateral meniscus had a mean posterior translation of

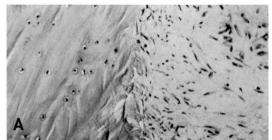
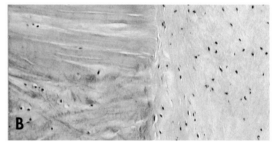
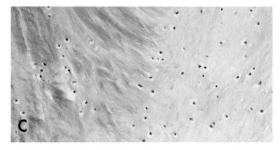

FIGURE 19
Photomicrographs of a fibrin clot-filled defect in the avascular zone of a canine medial meniscus at **(A)** 1, **(B)** 3, and **(C)** 6 months. Note the maturation of the repair tissue in the absence of a blood supply. (Reproduced with permission from Arnoczky SP, Warren RF, Spivak J: Meniscal repair using an exogenous fibrin clot: An experimental study in dogs. *J Bone Joint Surg* 1988;70A:1209–1217.)

approximately 11.2 mm. Whereas posterior translation of both menisci occurred throughout the range of motion, it appeared minimal between 15° and 60° of flexion. Extremes of motion (flexion and extension coupled with internal or external rotation) also cause marked alterations in the normal configuration of the menisci.[70] Although extremes of motion may place additional stress on the repaired meniscus (depending upon the location and extent of the injury), an experimental study has shown immobilization is detrimental to meniscal repair[71] by decreasing collagen formation and maturation.

WEIGHTBEARING

Weightbearing (compressive) forces are translated into tensile forces as a result of the structure and design of the menisci. These tensile forces (sometimes referred to as hoop stress), which tend to expand the menisci, are held in check by the collagen architecture of the meniscus and the firm attachments of the anterior and posterior horns of the menisci to bone. Although weightbearing would tend to compress the edges of a vertical, longitudinally oriented peripheral tear, it would tend to separate the edges of a transverse radial tear. Because most meniscal repairs involve longitudinally oriented peripheral tears, it would appear that early weightbearing should not have an adverse effect on healing in this group of repairs.

INDICATONS FOR MENISCUS REPAIR

Whenever a meniscus tear is encountered, the surgeon should initially assess whether it can be repaired, left alone, or excised. There are multiple factors to consider when making this decision, including tear type, associated anterior cruciate ligament (ACL) tear, patient age, chronicity of the tear, medial versus lateral meniscus, the presence of secondary tears, and others. The ideal type of tear for repair is vertical longitudinal within the peripheral 3 mm and the red-red and red-white zones. Tears with rim widths of 4 to 5 mm can still be successfully repaired, especially in conjunction with an ACL

reconstruction, even in patients as old as 55 years. Tears of that size in ACL-stable knees probably should be excised if the patient is older than 45 to 50 years. Because of the rich blood supply in the posterior horn origin of the lateral meniscus, complex tears in this location should be considered for repair if ACL reconstruction is to be done. Radial split tears in the posterior horns can be repaired using a purse-string suture technique (described later) when ACL reconstruction is to be done. Radial split tears of the middle third of the lateral meniscus do poorly when repaired, and may be better off left alone (Fig. 20) or minimally trimmed. In general, most flap tears are not amenable to repair unless located at the posterior horn origin of the lateral meniscus. There appears to be no benefit in trying to repair horizontal cleavage tears. Lateral meniscus repairs do better than medial meniscus repairs, and hence lateral meniscus tears have broader indications for repair. For example, a 50-year-old with a torn posterior horn of the lateral meniscus and an intact ACL has a better chance of successful repair than a 40-year-old with a tear of the posterior horn of the medial meniscus. Certain tears can be left alone, especially in a knee about to undergo ACL reconstruction, which would decrease the stress on the posterior horn of the medial meniscus.[60] Short tears less than 1 cm can be left alone, as well as incomplete tears that do not subluxate into the joint more than 3 mm on probing (Fig. 21). Fitzgibbons and Shelbourne[72] promote

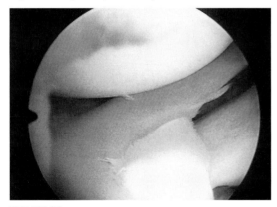

FIGURE 20
An example of a "leave alone" tear: this radial split tear of the middle third of the lateral meniscus can be left alone, or minimally trimmed. Meniscal repairs of the middle third of the lateral meniscus heal poorly. (Reproduced with permission from Primal Pictures, London, England)

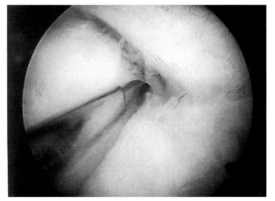

FIGURE 21
Another example of a "leave alone" tear, this being a 1-cm tear in the middle third of the lateral meniscus, and asymptomatic.

leaving alone stable posterior horn tears of the lateral meniscus in knees undergoing ACL reconstruction. They encountered no symptomatic failures in 189 lateral meniscal tears followed up for an average of 2.6 years after ACL reconstruction.

TECHNIQUES OF MENISCUS REPAIR

There are 3 basic types of repair: the inside-out, outside-in, and the all-inside technique. The inside-out technique can be further subdivided into the double-barrel cannula and single-needle passage techniques. Double-barrel systems predispose the surgeon into placing horizontal mattress sutures. Because collagen bundles are oriented predominantly circumferentially on the periphery of the meniscus, Asik and associates[73] and Rimmer and associates[74] found that a vertically oriented suture will secure more of these bundles than a horizontally placed suture and hence provides greater resistance against pullout. The former group also found that the weakest technique was knot-end sutures.

Thus, a double-barrel system may be more prone to suture pullout, or it may not provide adequate meniscal coaptation (Fig. 22), unless it is used as a single-barrel system by rotating it between needle throws to create vertically oriented sutures (Fig. 23). Most surgeons use nonabsorbable suture material because of its better strength over the initial 2 to 4 months. Barrett and associates,[75] in a clinical study, showed that permanent suture was better than absorbable suture in that it provided for longer and more stable fixation, permitting more complete maturation and remodeling of the meniscus. Eggli and associates[76] also reported better healing rates using nonabsorbable sutures.

Abrasion of the tear site and adjacent synovium is now the standard of treatment. Trephination of the rim may play a role in certain cases based on the work of Zhang and associates,[77,78] who demonstrated that patients treated with trephination and suturing had fewer symptoms and lower clinical failure rate compared to patients whose meniscal tears were treated with suturing alone.

They also showed the advantage of trephination in a goat model. Fox and associates[79] reported good results of trephination of incomplete meniscal tears without suturing.

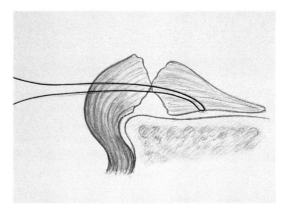

FIGURE 22

Double-barrel needle passes may create poor coaptation at the tear site as well as a greater chance of suture pullout. Drawing courtesy of Jeanne Koelling. (Reproduced with permission from Cannon WD: Arthroscopic meniscal repair, in McGinty JB (ed): *Operative Arthroscopy*. New York, NY, Lippincott-Raven Press, 1991, p 238.)

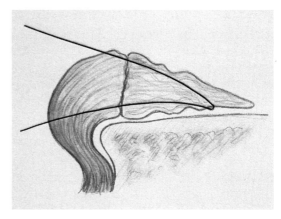

FIGURE 23

Using 2 separate needle passes, the surgeon can create a divergent suture containing enough meniscal tissue to provide excellent coaptation at the tear site. Drawing courtesy of Jeanne Koelling. (Reproduced with permission from Cannon WD: Arthroscopic meniscal repair, in McGinty JB (ed): *Operative Arthroscopy*. New York, NY, Lippincott-Raven Press, 1991, p 238.)

INSIDE-OUT REPAIR

Henning Technique of Meniscus Repair

Medial Meniscus Repair Although this technique was the first one used in North America, it is still an excellent technique, giving perhaps greater flexibility in repairing complex tears compared to other techniques. The most commonly cited disadvantage of the Henning technique is the greater degree of difficulty in needle retrieval of the 2.5-in needles compared to techniques using long needles.

Cannon has described his modification of the Henning technique.[80,81] A tourniquet is placed around the proximal thigh but is rarely used. It is therefore important to resist the temptation to resect synovium that may be partially obstructing the view anteriorly in the joint unless there is no other choice. Otherwise, bleeding may interfere with visualization throughout the surgery. If ACL reconstruction is to be carried out at the same time, tourniquet use may be necessary then, but ACL reconstruction still can easily be done without the use of a tourniquet. A well-padded leg holder is placed under the proximal thigh just distal to the tourniquet, and when meniscal repair is to be carried out, the thigh should be elevated approximately 35° to 40° in the leg holder to gain access to the posteromedial or posterolateral corner of the knee (Fig. 24). It is important to pad the leg holder well and place it on the thigh just distal to the tourniquet to prevent any pressure posteriorly on the sciatic nerve. Elevation of the thigh may not be necessary if the surgeon prefers to sit and flex the end of the table, but the thigh must extend far enough beyond the edge of the table break for the surgeon to gain access to the posterior corners of the knee. The leg may be kept in this position without redraping if ACL reconstruction is to be carried out after meniscal repair. The well leg should also be protected to prevent well leg palsies from occurring.

The surgeon's index of suspicion should be such that the leg is positioned appropriately for meniscal repair before arthroscopic inspection is done. Inspection should always include the pos-teromedial compartment. This is accomplished from the anterolateral portal by penetrating the triangular space bordered by the posterior cruciate ligament, the lateral border of the medial femoral condyle, and the superior surface of the posterior horn of the medial meniscus (Fig. 25). Probing the posterior horn of the medial meniscus while viewing from this position will allow the surgeon to better characterize the primary tear, and to identify secondary and tertiary tears of the posterior horn (Fig. 26).

After diagnostic arthroscopy has established a reparable meniscal lesion, a 6-cm longitudinal incision is made in the soft spot between the posterior border of the medial collateral ligament and the posterior oblique ligament (Fig. 27). Because needles penetrating the posterior horn of the medial meniscus tend to dive distal to the joint line, two thirds of the incision should lie below the joint line, one third above. If the arthroscope from the anterolateral portal is left in the posteromedial compartment, the arthroscope's light spot should help the surgeon identify and not cut the saphenous vein, which lies close to the incision. If the knee is flexed, the pes anserinus and the sartorial branch of the saphenous nerve will lie posterior to the joint line, but care must be taken throughout the procedure to avoid excessive

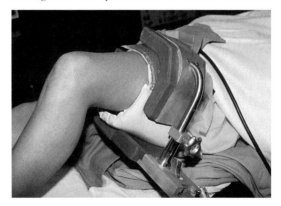

FIGURE 24
A thigh holder placed distal to the tourniquet and well padded posteriorly flexes the thigh up 45°, providing excellent access to the posteromedial and posterolateral corners of the knee. (Reproduced with permission from Cannon WD: Arthroscopic meniscal repair, in McGinty JB (ed): *Operative Arthroscopy.* New York, NY, Lippincott-Raven Press, 1991, p 238.)

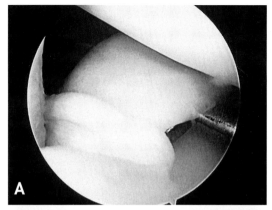

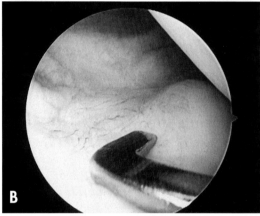

FIGURE 25

A, The posteromedial compartment should be inspected by passing the arthroscope from the anterolateral portal, either under direct vision, or with a blunt obturator in the sheath, through the triangular space bordered by the medial femoral condyle, the superior surface of the medial meniscus, and the posterior cruciate ligament. The probe is put under the posterior horn origin of the medial meniscus for easy retrieval when the surgeon is viewing posteromedially. **B,** The meniscosynovial junction of the posterior horn of the medial meniscus is clearly seen and probed from this vantage point.

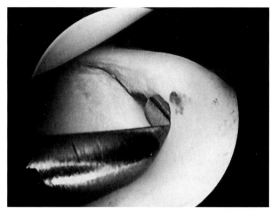

FIGURE 26

This incomplete vertical longitudinal tear of the posterior horn of this left medial meniscus was hard to see from the standard anterior viewing spot, but easily seen and characterized by passing the arthroscope through the triangular space described in Figure 25.

retraction or entrapping the nerve with sutures. As dissection is carried down to the posterior capsule, the surgeon should palpate for the direct head attachment of the semimembranosus to the posterior tibial tubercle. This is a key and easy landmark to feel. The surgeon should try to dissect anterior to this insertion, but not penetrate the posterior capsule. If it is inadvertently nicked, suture it closed.

If the direct head of the semimembranosus is too tight and too close to the joint line to make needle retrieval easy, it may be necessary to release several millimeters of its attachment. However, this is rarely necessary. If a tear longer than 2.5 cm is to be sutured, then subcutaneous tissue should be dissected off the superficial surface of the medial collateral ligament anterior to the posteromedial incision to accommodate needle retrieval. Because needle retrieval can be the most time-consuming part of meniscal repair, take enough time to create good exposure when making the posterior incision.

A popliteal retractor is inserted through the posteromedial incision behind the posterior capsule. The retractor may be one of those that are commercially available, such as the one designed by Charles Henning (Fig. 28), or improvised by using one half of a pediatric vaginal speculum, or even using a small spoon. A joint distractor occasionally is used for repairing tears of the medial meniscus longer than 2.5 cm in tight medial compartments because this will improve visualization when multiple sutures are to be used. A 3/16-in Steinmann pin is placed just proximal to the adductor tubercle and a second in the anteromedial flair of the tibia. The joint distractor is applied, and the medial compartment opened up (Fig. 27). If this does not allow adequate visualization of the posterior horn of the medial meniscus, Henning

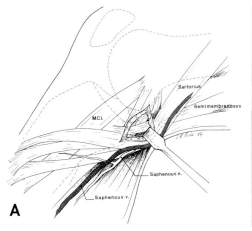
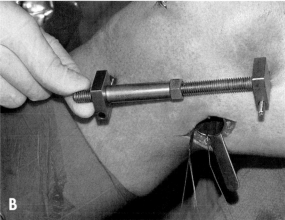

FIGURE 27
A, The posteromedial approach for retractor placement and needle retrieval. (Reproduced with permission from Brown GC, Rosenberg TD, Deffner KT: Inside-out meniscal repair using zone-specific instruments. *Am J Knee Surg* 1996;9:144–150.) **B,** A knee distractor is used for medial meniscal repairs. This enables better visualization of the posterior horn. The popliteal retractor can be seen in the posteromedial incision. (Reproduced with permission from Cannon WD: Arthroscopic meniscal repair, in McGinty JB (ed): *Operative Arthroscopy.* New York, NY, Lippincott-Raven Press, 1991, p 239.)

(personal communication, Wichita, KS, 1985) has suggested making multiple staggered transverse stab incisions in the medial collateral ligament between the medial joint line and its origin at the medial epicondyle in order to gain an additional 2 to 4 mm of joint opening. Cannon has used this technique to reduce displaced bucket-handle tears of the medial meniscus that otherwise were not reducible and would have been excised. Also, partial release will improve visualization of the posterior horn of the medial meniscus in patients with tight medial compartments.

Since 1983, when Henning suggested that rasping of the perimeniscal synovium and tear site might improve neovascularization and hence healing,[34,65] rasping has been done on all chronic and most acute repairs. Digital palpation posteromedially or posterolaterally to identify a tentative site of introduction followed by insertion of a spinal needle through the synovium in the posteromedial incision (Fig. 29) will determine the optimal site for insertion of 2- and 3-mm rasps (Fig. 30). The ideal site should be close to the plane of the superior surface of the posterior horn of the meniscus. Perimeniscal synovial abrasion is then carried out under direct vision over the superior portion of the peripheral rim of the meniscus to the tear site.

Both sides of the tear site should be freshened, especially if the tear is older than 8 weeks. A right angled rasp is helpful in accomplishing this. Henning and associates[82] have shown improved results when the bucket-handle side of the tear is rasped. In Figure 31, Henning took a biopsy of the handle side of a bucket-handle tear and showed a buildup of amorphous debris, an impediment to healing. A biopsy of the rim side of the same tear

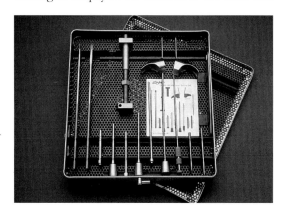

FIGURE 28
The Henning meniscal repair set consists of 2 rasps, a needle holder, a joint distractor, and a variety of cannulas. (Reproduced with permission from Cannon WD: Arthroscopic meniscal repair, in McGinty JB (ed): *Operative Arthroscopy.* New York, NY, Lippincott-Raven Press, 1991, p 238.)

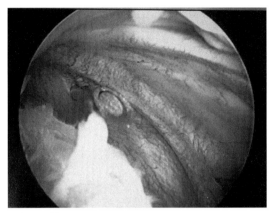

FIGURE 29
A spinal needle introduced through the soft spot at the pos-teromedial corner of this left knee will assure accurate orien-tation for rasping tears of the posterior horn of the medial meniscus.

showed a clean layer of fibrochondrocytes with-out amorphous debris, a more ideal condition for meniscal healing. The inferior surface of a poste-rior horn tear as well as the superior and inferior surfaces of a midcentral tear are best rasped with a burr type rasp or edge-cutting rasp introduced anteromedially. It is important to devote enough time to adequately abrade the tear site and sur-rounding synovium, both on the superior and inferior surfaces of the meniscus.

With the surgeon applying a moderate valgus force to the 20° to 30° flexed knee, suturing of the posterior horn origin of the medial meniscus is initiated. Sutures are 2-0 nonabsorbable Ethibond [Johnson & Johnson, Inc., Ethicon Div., Somerville, NJ (Special order D-6702)] with 2.5-in double-armed taper-ended Keith needles. A 10° to 15° bend is made 4 mm from the needle tip and a second 10° to 15° bend in the same direc-tion is made approximately 10 mm from the first bend (Fig. 32). These 2 bends are most easily made with a needle holder. The needle is then press-fit loaded into the needle holder (Stryker Corporation, Kalamazoo, MI).

Sutures for the posterior horn of the medial meniscus are placed from the anteromedial por-tal. A short cannula is placed through the antero-medial portal close to the medial edge of the patellar tendon and just over the superior surface of the anterior horn of the medial meniscus.

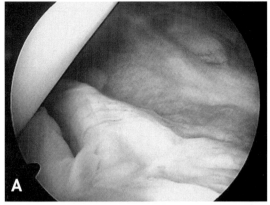

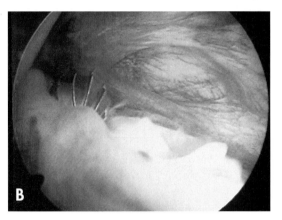

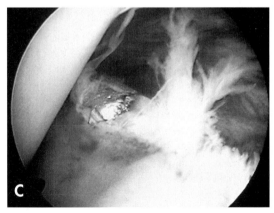

FIGURE 30
A, This chronic tear of the posterior horn of the left medial meniscus has rounded edges and unless freshened and abraded will not heal well after suturing. **B,** A 2-mm burr has been introduced from the posteromedial side and is being used to abrade the tear site. **C,** A 3-mm flat rasp has been introduced from the posteromedial side and is further abrad-ing the tear site.

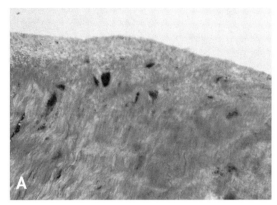

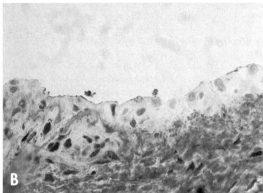

FIGURE 31
A, A biopsy from the handle side of a bucket-handle tear shows amorphous debris buildup, a potential barrier to healing. This material must be abraded off. **B,** A biopsy from the rim side of a bucket-handle tear shows fibrochondrocytes at the tear site and no debris. This condition is more conducive to healing. (Photomicrographs courtesy of Charles E. Henning, MD.)

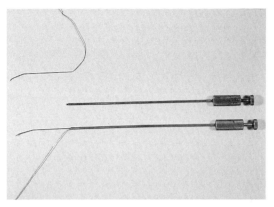

FIGURE 32
Double armed 2½-in Keith needles are bent approximately 15° twice and press fit loaded in the Henning needle holders. The suture is 2-0 Ethibond [Johnson & Johnson, Inc., Ethicon Div., Somerville, NJ, (Special order D-6702)].

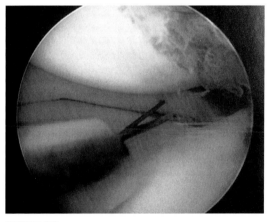

FIGURE 33
The first suture is being placed through the inferior surface of this left medial meniscus from an ipsilateral portal, making the suture more radially oriented across the tear site and hence stronger.

When suturing the majority of vertical longitudinal tears of the posterior horn, suturing is begun close to the posterior horn origin of the tear. However, in cases of displaced bucket-handle tears, it is at times preferable to place the first suture at the midpoint of the bucket-handle fragment, then to repair the posterior segment followed by the anterior segment, thus providing more accurate coaptation of the fragment to the remaining rim.

When starting at the posterior horn origin, the first suture preferably should be placed on the inferior surface of the meniscus followed by one on the superior surface (Fig. 33). Once the needle has been inserted approximately 3 to 4 mm from the tear site and up to the second bend in

the needle, a third bend in the needle is created by pushing the cannula and needle holder into the intercondylar notch (Fig. 34). The extra bend in the needle directs the needle away from the middle of the popliteal fossa and allows easier needle retrieval from the posteromedial incision. The importance of this third bend in the needle cannot be overemphasized. Further penetration of the meniscus is done with the needle holder in the intercondylar notch, otherwise the needle will exit either through the direct head of the semi-

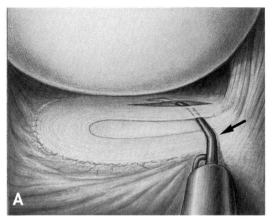
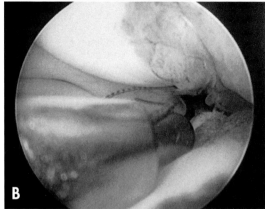

FIGURE 34

A, The first suture placed close to the posterior horn of either medial or lateral meniscus can be difficult to retrieve posteriorly. Hence, a third bend in the needle is made by levering the cannula and needle holder into the intercondylar notch. The additional bend in the needle will allow the surgeon to guide the needle into the popliteal retractor with greater ease. Drawing courtesy of Jeanne Koelling. (Reproduced with permission from Cannon WD: Arthroscopic meniscal repair, in McGinty JB (ed): *Operative Arthroscopy.* New York, NY, Lippincott-Raven Press, 1991, p 240.) **B,** The cannula with accompanying needle holder are levered into the intercondylar notch, thus creating a third bend in the needle so that it can be more easily retrieved at the posteromedial incision.

membranosus, or midline to it. This first suture throw should be directed from the inferior surface upwards through the meniscus so as to include as much meniscal tissue in a vertical orientation as possible. The surgeon may then carefully palpate the posterior capsule to determine whether the exit site of the needle will allow it to be retrieved from the posteromedial incision with or without the popliteal retractor in position. Frequently needles may be retrieved without the popliteal retractor in place, especially if the needles are heading more proximally or distally than the area contained within the popliteal retractor.

The surgeon should flex the knee to 45° to 55° to make posteromedial needle retrieval easier by relaxing the posterior structures and improving visualization. Once the point of the needle, which should be medial to the direct head of the semimembranosus, has been identified, the needle may then be advanced and grasped with the needle holder (Fig. 35). To prevent fingerstick injuries from the point of the needle, the needle should never be advanced while palpating posteriorly. The use of tapered-ended rather than trochar-ended needles definitely decreases the risk of finger puncture. After

release of the needle anteriorly, it is pulled out through the posteromedial incision. The second throw of the first suture should penetrate peripheral to the tear site near the meniscosynovial junction, creating a vertically oriented suture (Fig. 33). In an alternate and less preferable suturing technique, the second throw of the suture is made horizontally approximately 3 to 4

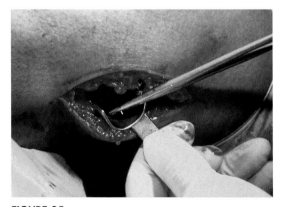

FIGURE 35

Once the tip of the needle has penetrated the posterior horn and capsule, it is deflected off the popliteal retractor and is retrieved with a needle holder. (Reproduced with permission from Cannon WD: Meniscal repair: The Henning technique. *Tech Orthop* 1993;8:95.)

mm from the first throw, thus creating a horizontal mattress suture. The needles should be passed in divergent directions so as to include as much meniscal tissue in a vertical orientation as possible (Fig. 36).

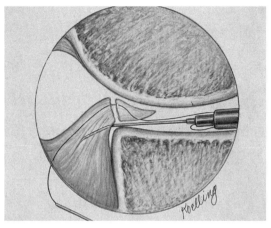

FIGURE 36
This diagram demonstrating the Henning technique shows excellent suture placement in the posterior horn with vertically divergent passes of the 2 needles. Note that one pass of the suture is close to the superior surface of the meniscus, and the second pass is underneath the inferior rim and penetrates through the meniscosynovial junction. Drawing courtesy of Jeanne Koelling. (Reproduced with permission from Cannon WD: Arthroscopic meniscal repair, in McGinty JB (ed): *Operative Arthroscopy.* New York, NY, Lippincott-Raven Press, 1991, p 240.)

The commonest suturing technique starts at the posterior horn origin, with suture placement alternating between the inferior and superior surfaces of the meniscus, spaced approximately 3 mm apart (Figs. 37 and 38). A better suturing technique, although more time consuming, is to stack the sutures on top of each other, with each suture containing approximately half of the thickness of the meniscus tissue (Fig. 39). Henning claimed improved healing rates using stacked sutures in contrast to fully divergent sutures.

If the tear extends into the middle third of the medial meniscus, the arthroscope should be switched to the anteromedial portal, and suturing should be done through the anterolateral portal (Fig. 40). An attempt should be made to direct the needles to the posteromedial incision site by bringing the needle holder anterior in the joint. The most anterior sutures may, at times, be directed out through a 1-cm incision placed between the posteromedial and the anteromedial incisions, but the suture knots usually will be palpable postoperatively (Fig. 41). Sutures placed in this fashion will avoid the shear forces that may result from sutures directed obliquely out through the posteromedial incision. If difficulty is encountered in adequately visualizing the posterior horn fragment, or if the suture needle tends to skive through the superficial layer of the meniscus, pro-

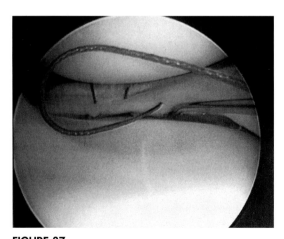

FIGURE 37
Vertically oriented sutures are placed approximately 3 to 4 mm apart, alternating between the superior and inferior surfaces of the meniscus.

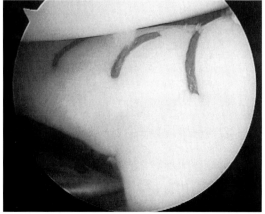

FIGURE 38
Three vertically oriented sutures are seen on the superior surface of the meniscus.

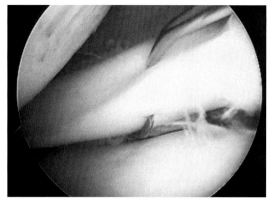

FIGURE 39
Technique of stacking sutures. Each vertically oriented suture secures approximately half of the thickness of the meniscus.

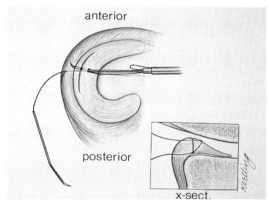

FIGURE 40
This diagram shows the technique for repairing the middle third of the medial meniscus. The arthroscope has been moved to the anteromedial portal, and suturing is carried out through the anterolateral portal. Note again the divergent needle placement, creating excellent coaptation of the meniscus. Drawing courtesy of Jeanne Koelling. (Reproduced with permission from Cannon WD: Arthroscopic meniscal repair, in McGinty JB (ed): *Operative Arthroscopy*, ed 2. New York, NY, Lippincott-Raven Press, 1996, p 304.)

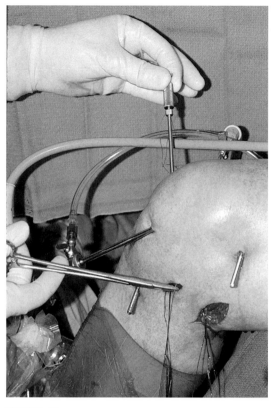

FIGURE 41
When suturing the middle third of the medial meniscus (as shown in Figure 40), occasionally a second incision may be made anterior to the posteromedial incision and sutures brought directly through this wound. These sutures have a more radial orientation than if they had been brought through the posteromedial incision. The knee distractor has been temporarily removed. (Reproduced with permission from Cannon WD: Arthroscopic meniscal repair, in McGinty JB (ed): *Operative Arthroscopy*, ed 2. New York, NY, Lippincott-Raven Press, 1996, p 304.)

viding weak fixation, it is very useful to introduce a probe through an accessory anteromedial portal made approximately 1 to 2 cm posterior to the anteromedial portal. The probe can be used to bring the meniscal fragment slightly anterior in the joint where needle penetration can be more easily achieved, or, more commonly, used to tilt the meniscus so that the angle of needle penetration into the meniscus is improved, thus securing more meniscal substance (Fig. 42). This technique is also valuable for aiding needle penetration through the inferior surface of the middle third segment of the medial meniscus. Occasionally, the needle will penetrate through the superior surface, but should not be redone because the resulting vertical suture provides excellent fixation.

The technique for repair of displaced bucket-handle tears is the same as that described above, once the bucket-handle fragment is reduced. Reduction is at times difficult, and may be aided

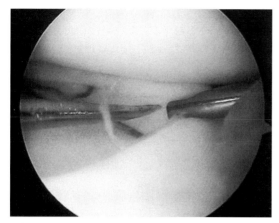

FIGURE 42
If difficulty is encountered in adequately visualizing the posterior horn fragment, or if the suture needle tends to skive through the superficial layer of the meniscus, providing weak fixation, it is very useful to introduce a probe through an accessory anteromedial portal made approximately 1 to 2 cm posterior to the anteromedial portal. The probe can be used to tilt the meniscus so that the angle of needle penetration into the meniscus is improved, thus securing more meniscal substance.

by applying a valgus force with the knee close to full extension. The application of a medial distractor allows the surgeon to control incrementally the amount of valgus force being applied to the knee. The 3/16-in pins will bend before the medial collateral ligament (MCL) will tear. In two cases, using the technique previously described, the MCL was partially released in order to reduce the bucket-handle fragment, and in another case, partial release of the MCL was necessary to visualize adequately the posterior horn tear of the medial meniscus. The MCL is partially released by retracting the posteromedial incision anteriorly and making 3 to 5 staggered transverse stab incisions with a number 15 scalpel blade, then applying more force with the medial distractor. When 2 to 3 mm of additional joint space has been obtained, the displaced meniscal fragment usually can be readily reduced. In the 3 cases mentioned above, none of the patients had any discernible residual MCL laxity.

If anterior cruciate ligament (ACL) reconstruction is to be performed, the sutures are not tied until the end of the reconstruction. The sutures can be kept tight during the ACL reconstruction

by threading them through 5- to 7-cm pieces of sterile intravenous extension tubing and cross-clamping the tubing to prevent damage to the suture material. This technique of Henning prevents redisplacement of a bucket-handle tear during the ACL reconstruction (Fig. 43). After the sutures are tied, the suture ends are not cut until the arthroscope is reinserted and the tear site probed to ascertain that the mobile fragment is well approximated to the rim. If 1 or more sutures are found to be loose, then these suture ends can be tied to adjacent suture ends, thus tightening the loose sutures and eliminating the need to completely replace the suture. Also, if the 2 ends of sutures are separated by too much soft tissue, the respective ends can be tied to other closer suture ends, thus reducing the risk of suture breakage postoperatively during knee motion.

Since Arnoczky and associates[38] showed that meniscal healing in the avascular zone of canine menisci occurred when fibrin clot was inserted into 2-mm punched-out defects in the meniscus, all isolated meniscal repairs have had fibrin clot introduced into the tear site before tying the sutures. Approximately 50 to 75 cm^3 of venous blood, drawn under sterile conditions by the anesthesiologist, is placed in a plastic container on the surgical field. The blood is stirred with

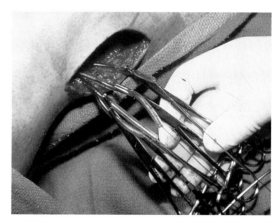

FIGURE 43
Threading intravenous tubing over the sutures and cross-clamping keeps the sutures organized and tight before tying them at the end of the case. (Reproduced with permission from Cannon WD: Henning technique for meniscal repair. *Tech Orthop* 1993;8:95.)

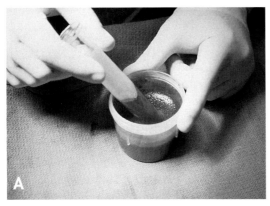
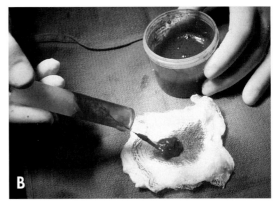

FIGURE 44
Fibrin clot is spun out of approximately 50 to 60 cm^3 of venous blood using a glass barrel from a syringe.

one or two 10- or 20-cm^3 glass syringe cylinders for approximately 5 to 10 minutes until the clot adheres to the glass cylinder(s) (Fig. 44). The clot is then removed and blotted with saline or Ringer's lactate moistened gauze. A suture (2-0 Ethibond) is placed at each end of the tubulated clot using 3 whip stitches (Fig. 45). After introduction of a 6- or 7-mm cannula, the 2 free needles are bent in the same manner as for meniscal repair and loaded into the Henning needle holders. They are then passed through the cannula 1 at a time under the inferior surface of the menis-

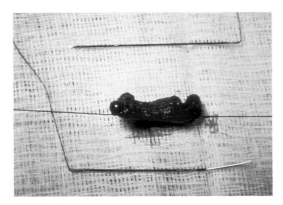

FIGURE 45
A 2-0 Ethibond suture (Ethicon) has been placed through each end of the fibrin clot to facilitate its stable placement under the inferior surface of the meniscus at the tear site. (Reproduced with permission from Cannon WD, Vittori JM: Meniscal repair, in Aichroth PM, Cannon WD (eds): *Knee Surgery: Current Practice.* London, England, Martin Dunitz, 1992, p 80.)

cus through the meniscosynovial junction at the posterior and anterior poles of the tear. They are retrieved posteriorly and tagged. The clot is both pulled through the cannula (Fig. 46) and pushed through using a blunt obturator. After the clot has been tucked into the tear site using a probe and/or Freer elevator, all sutures are tied. The single strands of the clot sutures are tied to adjacent meniscal repair sutures. Alternative methods of clot introduction include using less venous blood and cutting the clot into smaller segments. Henning preferred introducing the clot through a glass syringe with a blunt 13-gauge curved needle.[82] The tear site is then pulled open with a probe, and with the joint evacuated of fluid so that the clot does not float away, the clot is placed under the inferior surface of the meniscus throughout the length of the tear. The sutures are then pulled tight, trapping the fibrin clot, and tied.

Lateral Meniscal Repair The technique of lateral meniscal repair is similar to that of the medial meniscus repair. A 6-cm vertical incision is made at the posterolateral corner of the knee. A longitudinal incision is made in the deep fascia along the distal posterior margin of the iliotibial band, and with the knee flexed 90° the biceps is retracted posteriorly (Fig. 47). Using blunt and digital dissection, progress toward the midline of the knee, first identifying the posterolateral aspect of the femoral shaft, then palpating the anteriorly sit-

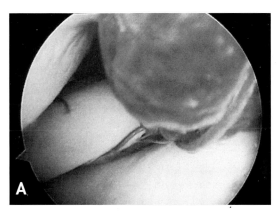 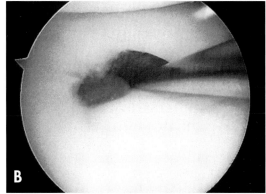

FIGURE 46
A, The fibrin clot is being both pushed with a blunt obturator and pulled with the previously placed clot sutures into the joint.
B, A Freer elevator is useful for tucking the fibrin clot under the meniscus.

uated lateral head of the gastrocnemius. Its muscle and tendinous origin is dissected off the posterior capsule, starting inferiorly and working in a superior direction to a point where a nerve hook passed from the anteromedial portal over the top of the posterior horn origin of the lateral meniscus can be palpated through the posterolateral incision. With the knee flexed 90°, the peroneal nerve will lie posterior to the biceps and need not be specifically identified. Although Henning used a joint distractor laterally, it is not necessary to use one. Abrasion of both tear surfaces is carried out as described for the medial side. All suture placement is done from the anteromedial portal, making it easier to direct the needle tips to the posterolateral incision for retrieval. It is more important to obtain ideal suture fixation at the posterolateral corner than to be too concerned if a suture passes through the popliteus tendon. The technique of fibrin clot preparation and introduction for isolated lateral meniscal tears in ACL-stable knees is the same as for the medial meniscus.

Radial split oblique tears of the posterior horn of the lateral meniscus close to its origin, a common tear pattern accompanying acute ACL tears, can be approximated with a pursestring suture made by passing 1 suture through the posterior leaf close to the inner edge of the meniscus, and the second throw of the suture through the anterior leaf of the tear close to the inner edge, then pulling it tight, approximating the edges of the

tear (Fig. 48). This tear pattern may be accompanied by a short vertical longitudinal component requiring additional sutures. Because adequate

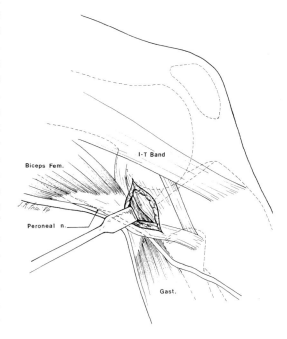

FIGURE 47
Posterolateral exposure for approaching the posterior horn of the lateral meniscus. (Reproduced with permission from Brown GC, Rosenberg TD, Deffner KT: Inside-out meniscal repair using zone-specific instruments. *Am J Knee Surg* 1996;9:144–150.)

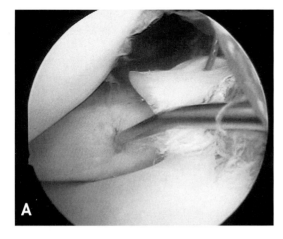

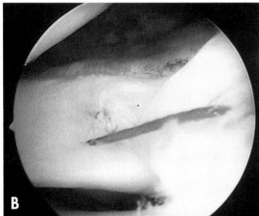

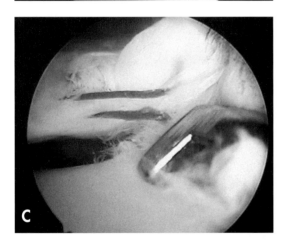

FIGURE 48
Two pursestring sutures are placed through the anterior and posterior leaves of this radial split-oblique tear close to the posterior horn origin of the lateral meniscus in this right knee.

healing has been difficult to achieve for radial split tears in the middle third of the lateral meniscus, they are probably best left alone, or minimally trimmed (Fig. 20).

More complex tear types, including oblique flap tears, broken bucket-handle tears, and missing meniscal segments, were repaired by Henning and associates[83] using fascial sheath fashioned from the fascia of the vastus lateralis and sutured superiorly and inferiorly over the torn meniscus. Fibrin clot is then injected into the sheath. Barrett and Treacy[84] also reported using fascial sheath to repair complex meniscal tears. Other surgeons do not appear to have adopted this difficult technique.

Complications of Henning Inside-Out Repair
Complications are surprisingly low in arthroscopic meniscus repair. Using the Henning technique, Cannon, in an unpublished series of 301 arthroscopic meniscal repairs, had 1 infection, 2 cases of thrombophlebitis, and 1 partial peroneal nerve palsy that resolved.

Rehabilitation of Henning Inside-Out Repair There are many different recommended rehabilitation techniques reported in the literature. Some recommend immediate full weightbearing and a full range of motion, whereas others recommend full weightbearing but keep the knee in an extended position. Others keep the patient nonweightbearing for up to 6 weeks with or without restricted range of motion. The final answer is not known, and almost any protocol that the surgeon wishes to follow is probably reasonable.

Cannon had previously recommended immobilizing isolated meniscal repairs at 20° to 40° of flexion for 3 weeks so that the fibrin clot had a better chance of remaining in the repair site.[81] However, current data recommend motion with or without weightbearing in order to prevent a significant reduction in meniscal collagen and aggrecan production,[71,85] and these latter findings may provide a good argument for commencing early motion after all meniscal repairs. Cannon still recommends nonweightbearing for the first 4 weeks, then partial to full weightbearing over the next

2 weeks. Then more aggressive closed kinetic chain activities are commenced. Running is started at 5 months, and some sports at 6 months.

Results of Henning Inside-Out Repair In Cannon's consecutive series of 301 patients that have undergone arthroscopic meniscal repair from 1982 until 1997, 172 were studied by either arthroscopic second look surgery or arthrogram for repairs of the medial meniscus. Henning's strict criteria for assessment of meniscal repair healing were used.[34] A meniscal repair was classified as healed if it had less than a 10% residual cleft at the tear site. If the cleft was less than 50% of the thickness of the meniscus, it was considered incompletely healed. If the residual cleft was greater than 50% of the thickness of the meniscus at any point over the length of the tear, it was classified as a failure (Fig. 49).

Seventy-eight percent of the meniscal repairs were associated with ACL reconstruction, and 22% were isolated meniscal repairs done in ACL-stable patients. The average age of the patients was 27 years. There were 59% medial and 41% lateral meniscal repairs. Sixty-seven percent of the repairs were chronic, done more than 8 weeks from the time of injury.

Of 172 patients who had an anatomic assessment of their healing, 70% had a satisfactory outcome (Fig. 50). (A satisfactory outcome is defined as the sum of the healed and incompletely healed menisci.) In the patients with ACL-reconstructed knees who underwent meniscal repair, satisfactory healing was obtained in 75%. In contrast, only 53% of the isolated meniscal repairs were considered to have a satisfactory outcome. This was highly statistically significant at the $p < 0.007$ level.

When these anatomic results were compared with clinical results, there was a marked difference. Patients were deemed to be clinically healed if they had no joint line pain or tenderness, clicking, or locking. Overall, 88% of the meniscal repairs were clinically healed (Fig. 51). In the ACL-reconstructed meniscal repair group, 92% were clinically healed, whereas in the isolated meniscal repair group in ACL-stable knees, 70% were clinically healed.

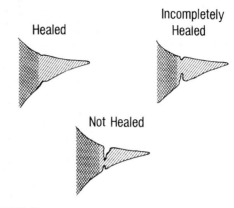

FIGURE 49
Six months after repair, the degree of healing can be determined by arthrogram for the medial side and arthroscopy for the lateral side. A meniscus is classified as "healed" **(A)** if it is healed over the full length of the tear with a residual cleft less than 10% of the thickness of the meniscus. A tear that is healed over its full length with a residual cleft that is less than 50% of its vertical height is classified as "incompletely healed" **(B)**. A residual cleft of greater than 50% of the thickness of the meniscus at any point over the length of the tear is classified as "failed" **(C)**. Drawing courtesy of Jeanne Koelling. (Reproduced with permission from Cannon WD: Arthroscopic meniscal repair, in McGinty JB (ed): *Operative Arthroscopy*. New York, NY, Lippincott-Raven Press, 1991, p 245).

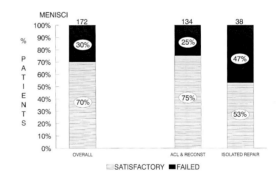

FIGURE 50
Meniscal repair results from second look arthroscopy and arthrography. Overall results are shown on the left side bar. The right 2 bars show a comparison of isolated repairs versus anterior cruciate ligament (ACL) reconstructions plus meniscal repairs. Successful outcomes (the sum of the healed and incompletely healed categories) of meniscal repairs associated with ACL reconstructions were 75%, in sharp contrast to 53% in the isolated repair group ($p < 0.007$).

Rim width and tear length were analyzed. There was better healing in patients who had 2-mm rim widths compared to patients with 4-mm or greater rim widths (Fig. 52). A similar relationship was found with tear length. Short tears healed better than long tears, such as a bucket-handle type tear (Fig. 53).

Lateral meniscal repairs did better than medial meniscal repairs (p = 0.11) (Fig. 54), although the difference was not statistically significant. Tears that were repaired within 8 weeks of injury did better than chronic tears repaired longer than 8 weeks from injury (p = 0.20) (Fig. 55). Interestingly, age of the patient did not appear to have an effect on meniscal healing (Fig. 56). There was no statistically significant difference in

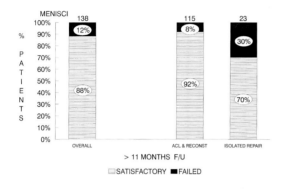

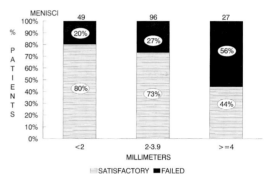

FIGURE 51
Meniscal repair results from clinical assessment. Overall satisfactory results were 88%. The right 2 bars show a comparison of isolated repairs versus anterior cruciate ligament (ACL) reconstructions plus meniscal repairs. Successful outcomes (the sum of the healed and incompletely healed categories) of meniscal repairs associated with ACL reconstructions were 92%, in sharp contrast to 70% in the isolated repair group.

FIGURE 52
Rim width versus healing. As meniscal rim width increases, the incidence of repair failure increases. (Figures 51–53, 56, and 57 are reproduced with permission from Van der Reis WL, Cannon WD: Arthroscopic meniscal repair using the inside-out technique: Anatomic and clinical follow-up. *Arthroscopy*, in press.)

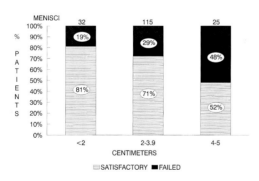
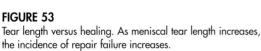

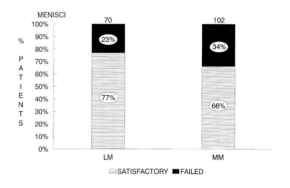

FIGURE 53
Tear length versus healing. As meniscal tear length increases, the incidence of repair failure increases.

FIGURE 54
Side of repair versus healing. Lateral meniscal repairs had an 77% satisfactory healing rate, whereas medial meniscal repairs were only 66% successful.

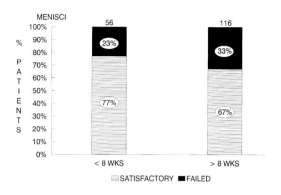

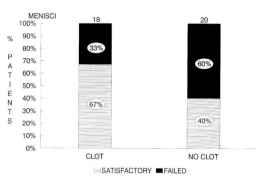

FIGURE 55

Time from injury versus healing. Repairs done less than 8 weeks from injury did slightly better than repairs done greater than 8 weeks from injury.

FIGURE 57

Use of fibrin clot versus healing. Although it would appear that the use of fibrin clot significantly increased successful healing, because of the small numbers the difference was not statistically significant ($p = 0.10$).

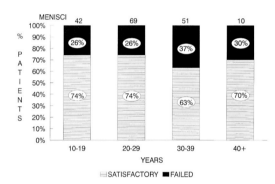

FIGURE 56

Age of patient versus healing. Age is not a deterrent to performing meniscal repair. Notice insignificant differences in the meniscal healing rate among the different age groups.

the satisfactory outcomes of patients in their second decade of life compared to patients in their fifth decade of life.

Repairs done in patients who reported a history of locking had only a 59% satisfactory healing rate, whereas patients who reported no history of locking had a 79% satisfactory healing rate ($p = 0.007$). The use of fibrin clot for isolated meniscal repairs in ACL-stable knees improved the healing rate (Fig. 57), but because of the small number of repairs, the results were not statistically significant ($p = 0.10$). Nevertheless, fibrin clot is still strongly recommended for use during isolated meniscal repair.

Inside-Out Repair Using Zone-Specific Technique

Rosenberg's group developed a single lumen curved cannula system (Concept, Largo, FL), which is versatile, allowing vertical or horizontal mattress placement through either the superior or inferior surface of the meniscus.[31,86,87] Currently this system uses 3 zone-specific cannulae curved to the right and 3 curved to the left (refers to the direction of the curve, not the side of the knee) (Fig. 58). Ten-inch needles with swedged on 2-0 nonabsorbable suture (Fig. 59) are passed 1 at a

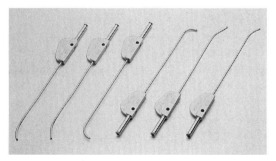

FIGURE 58

The zone-specific system uses 3 cannulae curved to the right and 3 curved to the left. (Courtesy of Linvatec, Inc.)

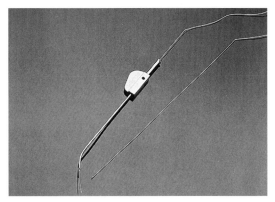

FIGURE 59
Ten-inch needles with swedged on 2-0 Ethibond are passed through the cannula. (Courtesy of Linvatec, Inc.)

time through the meniscus and safely away from the posterior neurovascular structures. When directed from the contralateral portal, the cannulae are designed to enable positioning with respect to the menisci, condyles, and tibial eminences. A major advantage of the zone-specific technique over other meniscal repair techniques is its ease of use and a short learning curve.

Indications for Zone-Specific Repair Repair of the meniscus begins with proper tear selection. Peripheral, unstable longitudinal tears (usually greater than 1.0 cm in length) without significant secondary components, and longitudinal tears within 3 mm of the periphery (red-white zone) are routinely repaired. Tears 4 to 6 mm from the capsule (white-white zone) are sometimes repaired, especially in younger patients undergoing ACL reconstruction. When repairing white-white tears or radial tears, the surgeon should consider supplementing the repair with insertion of a fibrin clot.

Flap tears, degenerative tears, and horizontal cleavage tears are not repaired. The surgeon should avoid the temptation to excise the peripheral components of double or triple bucket-handle tears. These can be repaired by including all of the components within multiple vertical sutures. With few exceptions, tears with rim widths ≥ 6 mm are not repaired.

There is no specific upper age limit for meniscal repair. Peripheral longitudinal tears of the lat-eral meniscus should be repaired in the patient older than 50 years. However, medial meniscus tears, unless at the meniscosynovial junction, are more apt to be treated by partial meniscectomy in this age group.

Brown and associates[87] do not routinely obtain preoperative arthrography or magnetic resonance imaging (MRI) to evaluate menisci for tears. MRI accuracy is probably 70% to 90%, better for the medial meniscus than the lateral. Both procedures can give the surgeon an estimated percentage chance that meniscal repair can be carried out. This is useful not only for the patient's preoperative planning, but also so that the surgeon can better plan his or her surgical schedule. From a medicolegal standpoint, it is advisable to discuss the possibility of meniscal repair with the majority of patients going into surgery with meniscal pathology. In order to cover the occasional meniscal repair done on a patient thought to be a candidate for partial meniscectomy, the consent should read "arthroscopy with probable meniscal surgery." Potential candidates are informed regarding the possibility of meniscus repair by reviewing the potential risks, benefits, and extended rehabilitation related to this procedure.

Important findings on the clinical examination are joint line tenderness, possible swelling, and occasionally a positive McMurray test. The McMurray test is performed in combinations of internal/external rotation and varus/valgus stress and carefully compared to the unaffected limb. A locked knee from a displaced bucket-handle tear is diagnostic in most cases, especially if unlocking is reported. Localized joint line pain with squatting or from hyperflexion provide further evidence of a meniscus lesion. A careful assessment for ACL deficiency, including arthrometer testing in suspicious cases is imperative because of its strong association with meniscal lesions.

Zone-Specific Repair Technique Brown and associates[87] prefer either general or epidural anesthesia for meniscal repair. The thigh muscles should be fully relaxed to allow an assistant to safely apply a varus or valgus stress for joint visualization and meniscal exposure.

Patient positioning must allow circumferential access to the affected knee during meniscus repair. The tourniquet and thigh holder are placed 12 to 14 in above the joint line. The patient is placed in the supine position so that the table break is just distal to the thigh holder, allowing access to the back of the knee and nearly complete flexion. A padded well-leg holder is used, and the unaffected limb is positioned in flexion, abduction, and external rotation. This arrangement increases the sterile field and facilitates the ease of needle passage and retrieval by the surgeon and assistant. Surgeons should wear water-resistant gowns that extend to the shoe tops to achieve a sterile field below the level of the patient's foot.

Diagnostic arthroscopy is performed with a 25° arthroscope, and the menisci are probed with a nerve hook to fully examine their superior and inferior surfaces. The probe is used to assess the type, location (vascularity), rim size, length, and stability of any tear encountered. The tourniquet may remain uninflated at this time to help assess vascularity. To expose the tear, the surgical assistant maneuvers the limb into various positions against the leg holder, controlling flexion while applying the desired amount of varus/valgus or rotational stress. The posterior horns and attachments of the menisci are viewed posteriorly through the intercondylar notch with a 70° arthroscope. An accessory posteromedial or posterolateral portal permits entry of a probe. A peripheral tear that can be viewed well within the posterior compartment is usually in proximity to blood supply and is a good candidate for repair.

Once the reparability of the torn meniscus is established, the tear zone and synovial fringes are prepared. Using a full-radius 4.5-mm curved motorized blade (Dyonics-synovator, Smith and Nephew Dyonics, Andover, MA) and/or a rasp, apposing margins of the tear are debrided of any fibrinous debris and synovium. This is especially important in chronic cases. Henning and associates[83] reported a reduced healing rate if tear site debridement was not performed. The motorized blade is also used to excoriate the perimeniscal synovium on the superior and inferior surface of the meniscus attachment beyond the tear site.

Most of the time the tear is posterior and peripheral, and a posteromedial or posterolateral portal is necessary for debridement and excoriation. The 70° arthroscope is again passed into the posteromedial or posterolateral compartment through the intercondylar notch. With the knee at 90° flexion, external digital palpation determines the approximate site for portal placement and an 18-gauge spinal needle is passed through the skin and capsule to identify the ideal site for the portal (usually 1 cm above the joint line and 1 cm posterior to the femoral condyle). The needle is removed and a small stab incision is made in the same spot with a #11 blade. Meniscal rasps or the 4.5-mm curved motorized blade can then be inserted posteriorly to prepare the meniscal tear and adjacent synovium.

In certain cases of stable tears, thorough preparation without suturing may be an optional "excoriation repair" in order to produce an acute healing response, usually in conjunction with ACL reconstruction. As a rule, surgeons do not create vascular access channels fearing compromise of the meniscal rim composed of circumferentially oriented collagen bundles.

Next, a posteromedial or posterolateral incision is made to facilitate retrieval of needles as they pass through the capsule, and to protect the neurovascular structures from injury. For the medial meniscus, a 3- to 4-cm incision is made posterior to the medial collateral ligament extending distally from the joint line. A common mistake is to position this incision too superiorly. The layer I aponeurosis is incised anterior to the sartorius permitting posterior retraction of the pes anserinus and sartorial branch of the saphenous nerve (Fig. 27, A). A combination of blunt and sharp dissection then allows direct palpation of the joint line sulcus. No attempt is made to dissect anterior to the semimembranosus or medial gastrocnemius tendons, which, like the capsule, are considered suitable for suture fixation. The exposure is completed by placing a retractor posterior to the medial head of gastrocnemius.

For lateral meniscal repair, the posterolateral incision is made posterior to the iliotibial band (ITB), extending 3 to 4 cm distally from the joint line, and separates the anterior aspect of the biceps femoris from the posterior margin of the ITB. Dissection is carried down anterior to the lateral head of the gastrocnemius and the arcuate complex and capsule, which lie anteriorly, then a retractor is inserted. This interval is easiest to develop 2 to 3 cm distal to the joint line where there is a more distinct tissue plane between the lateral head of the gastrocnemius and the capsule. The peroneal nerve lies medial to the biceps femoris and is not protected by retraction of the biceps alone. Rather, it is the retracted gastrocnemius that provides protection of the peroneal nerve during needle retrieval (Fig. 47). Sutures are tied against the posterolateral capsule, and are not tied over the muscle belly of the lateral head of the gastrocnemius.

Repair of the medial meniscus is done with the knee in relative extension (usually 5° to 15° flexion), which lines up the capsular rim side with the unstable side of the tear and avoids posterior capsular plication. The lateral meniscus is usually repaired with the knee flexed beyond 45°, which improves the needle retrieval space deep to the lateral gastrocnemius and also allows the peroneal nerve to drop further posteriorly. A retractor is inserted, and sutures are passed arthroscopically across the tear from "inside-out."

The zone-specific system includes 3 left and 3 right 2.7-mm cannulae, each set corresponding to the posterior, middle, and anterior zones of the meniscus. The cannulae are not malleable. However, for surgeons preferring a smaller and malleable set of cannulae, there is a set available commercially. The cannulae are prebent with a 15° up-curve near the tip to facilitate needle passage at the level of and parallel to the joint line. The curves of the cannulae accommodate the tibial eminences and condylar surfaces, allowing for positioning above or beneath the meniscus (Fig. 60). The needle tip is generally protruded slightly from the beveled portion of the cannula tip to allow for "harpooning" and reducing the unstable portion of the meniscus prior to passage across the tear. The beveled tip facilitates suturing on the inferior surface of the meniscus (Fig. 60, B). The posterior cannula may be positioned either posterior or anterior to the tibial spines. All repairs are done from the contralateral portal while viewing from the ipsilateral portal. Nonabsorbable suture (2-0 ticron or Ethibond) swedged to paired 10-in by 0.24 diameter straight needles is used in most cases. Second-look studies provide valuable information regarding the status of meniscal repair.[88,89] Rosenberg and associates[88] found that nonabsorbable sutures did not abrade or damage the articular hyaline cartilage and became thinly encapsulated or even broke after several months. Absorbable sutures may be acceptable for capsular tears, but longer lasting nonabsorbable sutures are generally required for tears within the body of the meniscus.

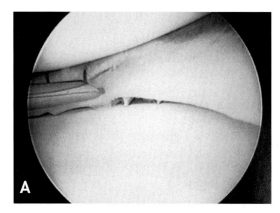
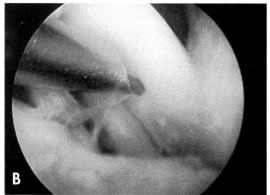

FIGURE 60
A, A zone-specific cannula is brought up against the superior surface of this right medial meniscal tear. Cannulae are always introduced from the contralateral portals. **B,** A cannula is used to place a suture through the inferior surface of the posterior horn of this left lateral meniscus.

The number and configuration of sutures depends on the type of tear and clinical judgment. Rosenberg and associates[86,87] use simple vertical or vertical mattress sutures and less frequently, horizontal mattress sutures placed at approximate 4- to 5-mm intervals on both upper and lower meniscal surfaces. Vertical sutures are alternated between superior and inferior surface of the meniscus, producing an anatomic reduction. For posterior horn tears, the anterior-most stitch usually is placed first as a reference for subsequent needle retrieval. Using the appropriate zone-specific cannula, the needle is advanced into the cannula until 2 to 3 mm of the needle point protrudes from the beveled tip. The point is then used to engage and reduce the meniscus fragment, after which the needle is advanced across the tear site and through the rim while an assistant views through the posterior incision. The needle is passed in small increments, 5 mm at a time, using a needle holder to secure the needle. This gives the assistant a better chance to retrieve the needle, preventing it from proceeding too far posteriorly and placing the neurovascular structures at risk. The needle should be contained by the posterior retractor. A needle holder then pulls the needle and attached suture out of the posterior incision.

The second needle at the other end of the suture is then passed to complete the stitch in an inside-out fashion. Because the single lumen cannula is low in profile, the second arm of the suture may be placed either in a vertical or horizontal fashion, but the vertical orientation is preferable because it is stronger (Fig. 61). Once again, the steps of needle passage described above are repeated, and the 2 suture ends of a pair are tagged with a clamp. Sutures are not tied until the repair and concomitant ligament surgery is complete. It is important to probe while lightly tensioning the sutures in order to assess reduction and stability. A minor "buckling" distortion of the meniscus is well tolerated and disappears during later knee motion. The sutures are tied over the capsular tissues, but if sutures exited the joint through the semimembranosus tendon, the medial head of the gastrocnemius, or the medial collateral ligament on the medial side, they are tied where they lie.

Two important points should be made. After thorough preparation of vertical longitudinal tears, repair is carried out to within 1 cm of the osseous posterocentral insertion. Suturing anterior to this point should be enough to reduce the meniscus, thus avoiding unnecessary difficulty or risk to the neurovascular structures. Ipsilateral suturing is not done. Medial tears are naturally apposed as the knee is extended secondary to the compressive effect of the medial femoral condyle. Secondly, in the lateral compartment it may be necessary to suture the unstable portion of the lateral meniscus to the popliteus tendon. Excoriation of the synovial covering of the tendon leads to proliferation of vascular tissue, which augments the healing process.

Fibrin clot is used for isolated longitudinal white-white tears, tears with a 4- to 7-mm rim in young patients with associated ACL reconstruction, and to supplement the repair of radial tears. In these cases, 60 cm³ of the patient's blood is obtained via phlebotomy and stirred with a glass rod in a glass syringe. After approximately 5 minutes of stirring, a well organized fibrin clot is formed in a "cotton candy" fashion. After gently washing its surface, the clot is removed from the glass rod and sutures are placed through it in a whip-stitch manner with 3-0 absorbable suture. The sutures left on each end of the clot are thread-

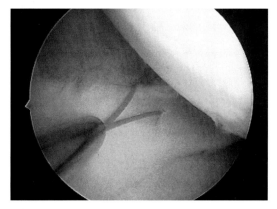

FIGURE 61
A vertically oriented suture is being placed in the middle third of the medial meniscus in this left knee.

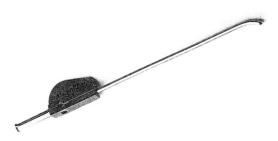

FIGURE 62
A slotted cannula is used to introduce fibrin clot into the tear site. (Courtesy of Linvatec, Inc.)

ed through a 10-in needle. The clot is then passed into the tear site using a slotted microcannula (Linvatec, Largo, FL) and the 10-in needle (Fig. 62). The sutures are directed through the anterior and posterior extent of the tear, and the clot is pulled gently into the tear site. The sutures are retrieved posteriorly in the same manner as the meniscus sutures and gently tied over the capsule. The slotted cannula design enables the surgeon to withdraw the small diameter cannula prior to pulling the clot through the anterior portal.

The clot can be further teased into the tear with the aid of a probe prior to final suture tying. The clot insertion into and onto the tear is achieved, hopefully sealing the zone from synovial fluid. Using a similar technique with the slotted microcannula, sutures with attached clot can be directed into the apex of a radial tear. With concurrent ACL reconstruction involving notchplasty and drilling of 2 tunnels, there should be adequate endogenous clot and hence exogenous fibrin clot is not prepared.

Rehabilitation of Zone-Specific Repair The knee is immobilized in a locked brace for 2 weeks. In young patients with large tears in the 4- to 6-mm avascular zone, immobilization is continued for 3 weeks. This period of immobilization is designed to keep the clot in position and maintain its integrity about the repair site before resuming motion. The degree of knee flexion that correlates with greatest apposition of the torn meniscus is assessed at arthroscopy, and the brace is locked

in that position. Usually this occurs at 10°. Occasionally it is necessary to modify the protocol with consideration given to the complexity of the meniscal repair, concomitant surgery, suture material, and so forth. Progressive weightbearing and range of movement exercises are commenced after 2 weeks. Squatting is avoided for 6 months. The rehabilitation of meniscal repairs done with concomitant ACL reconstruction generally follows the ACL protocol, but movement is restricted for the first 2 weeks.

Results of Zone-Specific Repair In Brown and associates' series,[87] 92% of selected peripheral tears (a rim size ≤ 3 mm) had clinically successful outcomes as defined by absence of signs and symptoms of a meniscal tear, return to high activity level, and lack of significant radiographic changes. Other studies have reported similar success rates, varying between 78% and 98.6%.[33,34,37,90,91]

Second-look arthroscopy, a more exact measure of anatomic healing, demonstrated that 24 out of 29 repairs were healed at a minimum of 3 months postoperatively. The other 5 were partially healed (30% to 50% healing), and 4 of these 5 were in ACL-deficient knees.[88]

Other Inside-Out Techniques

Another inside-out technique (Arthrex, Inc., Naples, FL) commercially available is economically cheap because it uses no special sutures and no swedged on needles. It comes with 2-mm cannulas that can be bent and shaped to fit through the joint to reach the torn meniscus. A cannula bender comes with the set of instruments. Because suturing is carried out from the contralateral portal, a bend is usually necessary to accommodate the tibial spines. The beveled tip of the cannula is used to help reduce and stabilize the most posterior part of the tear. A nitinol needle is then inserted with the help of a pusher and brought through the meniscus and out against a popliteal retractor that comes with the set (Fig. 63). Because this system uses nitinol needles, the needle tends to come out straight from the bent cannula, making retrieval easier. The needles may be reused, and a second pass with the needle is done next to the

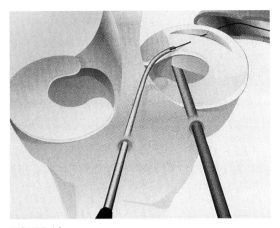

FIGURE 63
A nitinol needle is passed through a malleable cannula and penetrates the posterior horn of the medial meniscus. A popliteal deflector protects the neurovascular structures. (Drawing courtesy of Arthrex, Inc.)

first pass, creating either a horizontal or vertical suture. Although most surgeons prefer to use 2-0 suture size, up to #1 size suture can be inserted on the end of the nitinol needle. Although it is considerably cheaper, a minor disadvantage of the technique is that a doubled suture is brought through the meniscus with each pass rather than a needle with a swedged on suture. There is also some debate as to whether nitinol needles are better than standard needles.

This instrument set also comes with a needle catcher to be used through an arthroscopic poste-rior portal and cannula. The nitinol needle is introduced through the meniscus from an ipsilateral portal and as it penetrates through the posterior attachment of the meniscus, it is captured with the needle catcher (Fig. 64). By advancing the needle, it is brought out of the joint through the cannula. Adjacent sutures passed in this manner are then arthroscopically knot tied through the posterior cannula. Although of theoretical concern only, by placing the knots intra-articularly, capsular plica-tion can be avoided.

Clancy and Graf[29] introduced a double lumen cannula (Smith and Nephew, Acufex, Mansfield, MA) that allowed placement of horizontal mattress sutures in a relatively simple fashion (Fig. 65). This was the first instrumentation that permitted pas-sage of 2 needles with attached suture simultane-ously without repositioning the cannula, which has a small slit connecting the 2 lumens for pas-sage of the suture loop (Fig. 66).

Complications of Inside-Out Repair

Complications are surprisingly low in arthroscop-ic meniscus repair. In the Henning technique reported in this monograph, Cannon, in a series of 301 arthroscopic meniscal repairs, had 1 infec-tion, 2 cases of thrombophlebitis, and 1 partial peroneal palsy which resolved. Small reported an overall incidence of 2.4% in 3,034 meniscal repairs collected from a group of surgeons.[92]

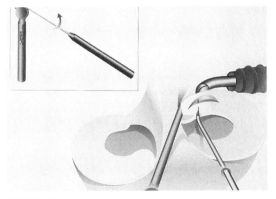

FIGURE 64
The same instrumentation as shown in Figure 63 except that a curved cannula retrieves the needles as they penetrate the pos-terior horn. Adjacent sutures are arthroscopically knot tied together through the cannula. (Drawing courtesy of Arthrex, Inc.)

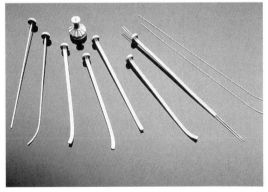

FIGURE 65
A double lumen slotted cannula instrument for placing hori-zontal sutures. (Drawing courtesy of Smith and Nephew, Acufex Microsurgical.)

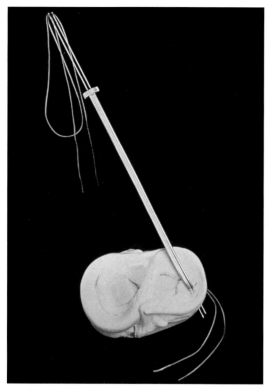

FIGURE 66
In this diagram, a horizontal suture is being placed through the posterior horn of the meniscus. (Courtesy of Smith & Nephew, Inc.)

These included 30 saphenous nerve injuries, 6 peroneal nerve injuries, 3 vascular injuries, and 11 deep infections. In contrast, Austin and Sherman[93] had an overall complication rate of 18% in 101 consecutive meniscal repairs. Popliteal artery injuries are most likely underreported. Stiffness has not been as much of a problem with isolated meniscus repair in ACL-stable knees as it has in meniscus repair with concomitant ACL reconstruction. Saphenous nerve injuries are more common, either severance of the infrapatellar branch of the nerve, or palsy by stretch or entrapment with a suture of the sartorial branch.[33,36,82,86] Stone and associates[94] reported a 10% incidence of transient saphenous nerve neurapraxias. Austin[95] stated that saphenous neuropathy is by far the most common complication after meniscal repair, and most patients describe it as being only a minor nuisance. Scott and asso-

ciates[34] reported 2 reoperations for broken parts of needles.

For meniscal repair using an inside-out technique with needles, most of these complications can be avoided with use of posterior incisions and popliteal retractors to protect the popliteal artery and vein, and the peroneal or saphenous nerves from injury.

OUTSIDE-IN TECHNIQUE

The advantage of the outside-in technique advocated by Warren[30] and others[81,96] is that it requires no specialized instrumentation other than an 18-gauge spinal needle and absorbable monofilament suture. Other advantages are that it is a rapid way of suturing a meniscus. It is particularly suited to the rare peripheral anterior horn tears, and attaching the anterior one third of meniscal allografts. Objections to the outside-in method include inadvertent hyaline cartilage injury from the unprotected needle tip, and difficulty suturing posteriorly.

Indications

The outside-in technique of arthroscopic meniscal repair was developed by Warren[30] as a method to decrease the risk of injury to the peroneal nerve during arthroscopic lateral meniscal repair. Because the starting point for needle entry is controlled, peroneal nerve injury is easily avoided during lateral meniscal repair. The outside-in technique can be used for repair of most meniscal tears. Tears in the anterior portion of the meniscus are easily accessed with this technique. In far posterior tears of the lateral meniscus, it may be difficult to start far enough posteriorly, thus resulting in oblique suture orientation across the tear. In this setting, the inside-out technique with a posterior incision may be preferable.

A significant advantage of the outside-in method is that sutures can be placed without the need for a large, rigid cannula for suture placement as is used for many inside-out techniques. Although there is a risk of causing minor damage to the articular surfaces when introducing needles from outside the joint, there is also risk of scraping the articular surfaces when using a rigid cannula in the inside-out technique. The outside-in technique also allows precise suture placement in areas of limited access because only small needles are used instead of the larger cannulas or needle holders used in the inside-out technique. This use of small needles can facilitate vertical suture placement. Except in very tight medial compartments, excellent visualization is possible because there are no instruments between the meniscus tear and the arthroscopic view. Finally, the repair can be performed with smaller incisions with less dissection than used with the inside-out technique.

The outside-in method can be used for suturing meniscal replacement (such as an allograft or synthetic device) to the capsule (Fig. 67). This method will also be useful for securing materials, such as a fibrin clot or a carrier containing growth factors, to a repair site. A suture can be placed across the tear, and then the implant or fibrin clot can be attached to the suture and brought into the tear site. Secure repair of meniscal tears or a meniscal replacement may often require a combination of methods, and thus the surgeon should be comfortable with several methods.

Technique of Outside-In Repair

The outside-in method requires only 18-gauge spinal needles, an arthroscopic grasper, and suture material.[97] Special instruments are also available, such as a wire cable loop for suture retrieval. The

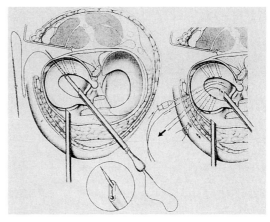

FIGURE 67
The outside-in technique can be used for suturing a meniscal allograft to the capsule. (Courtesy of Smith & Nephew, Inc.)

knee is placed into approximately 10° flexion for medial meniscus repair and 90° flexion for lateral meniscal repair to avoid peroneal nerve injury. While the surgeon is viewing the meniscus arthroscopically, the needle is placed across the tear site from the outside. The starting point is located by palpation and by using topographic landmarks. Transillumination may be used to identify small cutaneous nerves and veins. The needle passes across the tear in the meniscus and penetrates the inner segment of the meniscus. The needle then enters the joint on either the superior (femoral) or inferior (tibial) surface of the inner segment of the meniscus (Fig. 68). A small skin incision is made,

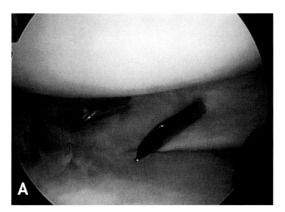
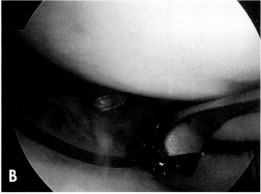

FIGURE 68
A, The spinal needle is placed across the meniscus tear from the outside, going across the tear and entering the joint on the tibial or femoral side of the inner segment of the tear. **B,** #0-PDS sutures are placed through the needle from the outside.

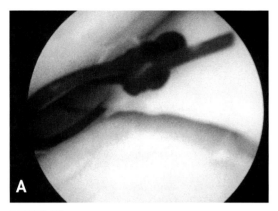
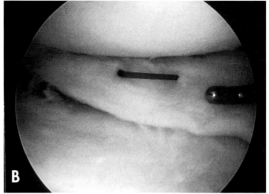

FIGURE 69
A, A mattress suture is created by tying adjacent sutures together outside the knee and then pulling the knot through the meniscus. **B,** The mattress suture reducing the meniscus tear.

and the subcutaneous tissue is spread down to the capsule. It is important to identify and protect the saphenous nerve and vein on the medial side.

A second needle is then passed, emerging from the meniscus adjacent to the first needle to achieve proper suture orientation. The second needle can be placed so as to create either a vertical or horizontal mattress suture across the tear. It is felt that a vertical suture orientation will more effectively capture the circumferentially-oriented collagen fibers of the meniscus. Suture (#0-PDS, Johnson & Johnson, Ethicon Div., Somerville, NJ) is next passed into each needle, grasped inside the joint, and pulled out the anterior portal. PDS suture is used because it is rigid enough to push through the needles. There are 2 ways to complete the repair: (1) Make a knot in the end of the suture with 3 or 4 throws in a standard square knot configuration. Then pull the knot back into joint so that the knot lies against the meniscus and maintains the tear in a reduced position. Then tie adjacent sutures together subcutaneously over the capsule. (2) Tie adjacent sutures together outside the anterior portal, using a standard square knot. Then pull the knot through the meniscus and tie the sutures together subcutaneously over the capsule. This technique allows creation of a mattress suture (Fig. 69). This procedure may be facilitated by placing a smaller "dilator knot" in front of the knot holding the 2 ends together, then pulling the sutures so that

this dilator knot passes through meniscus prior to the larger knot. The dilator knot is a square knot made with only 2 throws.

Another method for passing the suture after the needles are placed across the tear site is to pass a wire cable loop through 1 cannulated needle, place the suture through the other needle, then place the emerging suture into the wire loop (Fig. 70). The suture is then pulled through the meniscus creating a horizontal mattress suture. The wire cable loop and cannulated needle are pulled out together, because the doubled suture may not easily fit into the 18-gauge spinal needle.

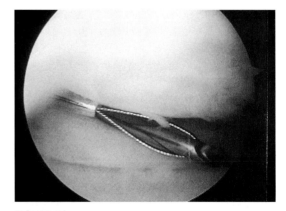

FIGURE 70
A wire cable loop is passed through one cannulated needle and a suture is placed through an adjacent needle. The emerging suture is then placed into the wire loop and pulled to the outside.

The advantage of this method is that it eliminates the need to pull the sutures out the anterior portal where the sutures may entrap soft tissue unless a cannula is used. This method also eliminates the need to pull the knot through the meniscus in order to make a mattress stitch.

It is also possible to use a permanent, braided suture with this technique. This is accomplished by passing a wire cable loop through the cannulated needle, then placing the end of the suture into the wire loop using an arthroscopic grasper inserted through the anterior portal. The suture is then pulled through the meniscus, after which the process is repeated with the wire loop to pass the other end of the suture through the adjacent needle.[98] The use of permanent suture may be preferable for repair of tears with poor healing potential, such as those in older patients, chronic tears, or tears with marginal vascularity.

Special Technical Considerations For Outside-In Repair

Careful attention to technique will aid in successful use of the outside-in method. Several other tips will also help to avoid problems and simplify the procedure. Needle placement across the meniscus may be made easier by using a probe or small loop curette to provide counter pressure on the meniscus during needle placement. It is helpful to place both needles across the tear site prior to passing the sutures in order to avoid the second needle cutting a previously placed suture. When pulling sutures out through the anterior portal, it is recommended to use a cannula in the anterior portal to avoid entrapment of soft tissue between the sutures. A 7-mm diameter arthroscopic cannula (Linvatec, Largo, FL) will allow passage of most standard arthroscopic grasping instruments. After 1 set of sutures has been placed, these sutures should be tied and pulled back into the knee before the next set of sutures is placed. This will avoid tangling of adjacent sets of sutures inside the knee.

Needle placement must remain anterior to the biceps tendon on the lateral side to avoid injury to the peroneal nerve. Curved needles (Smith and Nephew, Acufex, Mansfield, MA) may be used for posterior tears to decrease the need for a posterior starting point and thus decrease the risk of neurovascular injury. Valgus or varus load can be applied when placing sutures on the medial or lateral meniscus, respectively, in order to open the compartment and make needle placement easier. This will also approximate the capsule to the meniscus, thus aiding in accurate meniscal repair. Accurate needle placement may require access to the posterior joint line. For lateral repairs the knee may be placed into a "figure-of-4" position (flexion of the knee and external rotation of the hip). In this position, the lateral side of the knee can project over the edge of the table, providing access to the posterior joint line. For medial meniscal repairs, it is helpful to drop the foot of the table to allow access to the posterior joint line.

If the needle points down towards the tibial surface as it enters the joint, the suture will be difficult to pass into the joint because the needle will hit the tibial surface. This problem can be solved by using a probe passed through the anterior working portal to hold up the tip of the needle and thus allow easier passage of suture into the joint. The needle can also be manipulated from the outside to place the tip in a position that will allow easy passage of suture into the knee.

Vertical suture orientation may be preferable because it will capture more circumferential collagen bundles. This orientation is easily accomplished with the outside-in technique. It is also recommended to place sutures on both the tibial and femoral surfaces of the meniscus to allow for a more secure repair (Fig. 71). The use of permanent suture is recommended if delayed healing is suspected (older patient, poor vascularity, and so forth). It is important to abrade the tear surfaces prior to suture placement to remove any synovial covering or amorphous acellular debris accumulation, and to stimulate vascular ingrowth. This may be accomplished with a rasp, burr, or 3.5-mm fullradius resector. Consideration may also be given to abrasion of the synovium immediately adjacent to the tear to stimulate further vascularity, as well as to the use of fibrin clot to augment healing in isolated meniscal repairs (Fig. 72). Fibrin clot is used for most isolated meniscal repairs, especially

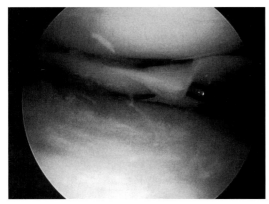

FIGURE 71
Sutures should be placed on both tibial and femoral sides of the meniscus to provide a secure repair.

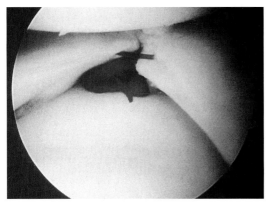

FIGURE 72
A fibrin clot may be placed at the tear site to augment healing of tears with poor healing potential due to marginal vascularity, underlying meniscal degeneration, or older patient age.

those tears with marginal vascularity. Fibrin clot is not necessary with concomitant anterior cruciate ligament (ACL) reconstruction because there is already a hemarthrosis from the ACL reconstruction. In the setting of concomitant ACL reconstruction, the meniscal repair sutures should be placed but not tied until the ligament graft is secured.

Complications of Outside-In Repair
With careful attention to surgical technique and local anatomy, complications are rare. Saphenous nerve injury can occur during needle passage on the medial side or if the sutures are inadvertently tied around the nerve or its branches. Careful dis-

section combined with transillumination will decrease this risk. Peroneal nerve injury will be avoided by performing lateral meniscal repair with the knee in 90° flexion and starting needle placement anterior to the biceps tendon.

Superficial infection may occur if careful soft-tissue coverage over the sutures is not achieved. A 2-layered wound closure over the sutures is recommended. Local acidity during degradation of absorbable sutures may contribute to the risk of infection. Aggressive early treatment of an infection usually will salvage the repair.

Limitation of extension may theoretically occur due to entrapment of the posterior capsule if the knee is in too much flexion while tying sutures that pass through the posterior capsule, especially on the medial side. This is quite unlikely to occur because during arthroscopic repairs the sutures are usually placed with valgus load applied to the knee, and in this position the capsule is closely apposed to the meniscus. This complication is probably more likely with open meniscal repair because the sutures are placed with the knee in flexion, a position in which the posterior capsule is lax, and could be accordioned into the sutures. The use of absorbable sutures will decrease the risk of permanent entrapment of the posterior capsule. Failure of healing can occur because of poor tear selection for repair (inadequate vascularity, degenerative tissue, and so forth), knee instability, inadequate suture stabilization of the tear, too oblique suture orientation across the tear, failure of early protection of the repair, and repeat injury. Careful attention to patient selection, surgical technique, and postoperative rehabilitation will minimize failure.

Rehabilitation of Outside-In Repair
Patients are placed into a hinged, double-upright brace for the first 6 weeks postoperatively. Early range of motion exercise is begun immediately, including full extension. Flexion is limited to 70° during the first 6 weeks to protect posterior horn repairs. Full weightbearing with the brace locked in full extension is allowed as tolerated. There does not appear to be any adverse effect on meniscal healing if ambulation is allowed in full

extension. The brace hinge is adjusted to allow a range of motion from 0° to 40° beginning at 4 weeks. Weightbearing out of the brace is allowed at 6 weeks. Running is begun at 4 months, with return to full athletic participation by 5 months. Squatting and hyperflexion are discouraged for up to 6 months following meniscal repair. In the setting of concomitant ACL reconstruction, the usual ACL rehabilitation protocol is used because this provides appropriate protection of the healing meniscus. The typical ACL rehabilitation protocol includes immediate full weightbearing in extension in a hinged brace. Progression to full range of motion is allowed immediately as tolerated, with emphasis on early achievement of full extension. At 3 to 4 weeks, the brace is unlocked to allow restoration of normal gait. Weightbearing out of the brace is allowed at 4 to 6 weeks. Closed kinetic chain strengthening exercises are begun in the second week and progressed. Sport-specific activities are initiated at 6 to 8 weeks for further development of strength and proprioception. Running is begun at 3 to 4 months with return to full athletic participation by 5 months.

Results of Outside-In Technique

The outcome was reviewed of outside-in meniscal repairs performed at The Hospital For Special Surgery (HSS) between 1984 and 1988.[99] Of 96 patients, six were lost to follow-up leaving a study group of 90 patients (74 males and 16 females). The minimal follow-up was 3 years, with an average follow-up of 46 months (range, 36 to 89 months). The average age was 25 years (range, 11 to 54 years). The interval from injury to repair averaged 11 months (range, 1 week to 11 years). Patients injured while participating in athletics made up 87% (78) of the total; 12 patients reported an insidious onset of symptoms.

The posterior horn of the meniscus was torn in 91% (82) of the group. The peripheral third of the meniscus was torn in 87% (78). There were 72 (80%) medial and 18 (20%) lateral repairs. An exogenous fibrin clot was used in 17 repairs in an attempt to augment healing.[100] Seven of the repairs in which the fibrin clot was used were located in the middle third of the meniscus (red-white region). All patients were evaluated with physical examination, radiographs, and objective evaluation of the meniscus with either computed tomography arthrogram, magnetic resonance imaging (MRI), and/or arthroscopic inspection. Four patients refused objective testing but underwent physical examination. The use of these objective outcome measures allowed more anatomic evaluation of the success of the healing process and excluded asymptomatic residual tears from the success group. Complete meniscal healing was determined by the absence of dye leaking into the tear site on the arthrogram, while partial healing was noted by intrusion of dye into 1 surface of the tear but without dye penetration to the other side of the tear. Failure of healing was noted by persistent dye throughout the entire thickness of the tear. MRI criteria for full healing include presence of low or moderate signal intensity at the tear site with complete apposition of the tear edges. Partial healing was noted on MRI by persistent high signal intensity but normal meniscal morphology at the tear site, while failure of healing was noted by high signal and abnormal meniscal morphology at the tear site.

Overall, 78 patients (87%) had a successful outcome. Sixty-two (69%) were asymptomatic and had objective evidence for complete healing of the meniscus (group I); 16 patients (18%) were minimally symptomatic and had objective evidence for partial healing (group II); and 12 patients (13%) had failure of healing (group III). These results indicate that the partially healed group II patients also had a satisfactory outcome.[99] There was a significant difference in healing rate between patients with a stable knee and those with an unstabilized ACL-deficient knee ($p < 0.05$). The failure rate was 38% (5/13) in unstable knees, 15% (5/33) in stable knees, and only 5% (2/38) in patients undergoing concomitant ACL reconstruction. (It is likely that the hemarthrosis that occurs during ACL reconstruction provides serum factors that aid meniscal healing.)

The failure rate was 15% (11/72) for medial meniscus repairs, compared to a 5% failure rate (1/18) for lateral meniscal repairs. Tears that involved the posterior horn of the medial meniscus had the highest failure rate, especially in the setting of ACL insufficiency. This is most likely due to the fact that the medial meniscus serves as a significant restraint to anterior tibial translation in the ACL-deficient knee. It is thus likely that in the ACL-deficient knee, the medial meniscus is exposed to higher shear stresses and thereby susceptible to injury. It is also possible that the higher failure rate for posterior tears was caused by oblique suture orientation across the tear, because this may occur using the outside-in technique.[101] Repairs failed more commonly in the central, less vascular portion of the meniscus. There was a 4% failure rate (1/23) for tears at the meniscocapsular junction compared to a 40% failure rate (4/10) for tears in the central third of the meniscus ($p = 0.02$).

There were 52 chronic and 38 acute repairs (defined as repair performed within 1 month of injury). There was no significant difference in the healing rate between these groups. The failure rate was higher for patients older than 30 years, although the difference did not reach statistical significance. There was a 12% failure rate (6/52) in patients younger than 30 years, compared to a 16% failure rate (6/38) in patients older than 30 years. The rate of partial healing, as compared to complete healing, was higher in the older age group. There was a 32% rate of partial healing (8/25) in patients older than 40 years.

Patients with an insidious onset of symptoms had a 66% rate of complete or partial healing, in contrast to a 90% rate of complete or partial healing in patients with traumatic onset. This difference suggests that there may be an element of underlying meniscal degeneration in patients with an insidious onset of symptoms. Such intrinsic degeneration may result in a lower healing potential.

There was a 36% failure rate (6/17) in tears in which a fibrin clot was used. Three of these failures were attributed to unrepaired ACL insufficiency and 3 were the result of complex tears in the avascular zone. Because the fibrin clot was used in tears with an inherently higher failure rate, no conclusions can be made regarding the efficacy of fibrin clot insertion. A randomized, prospective study is required to assess the efficacy of fibrin clot use in meniscal repair.

The complication rate was 3% (3/90). There was 1 superficial infection, 1 case of thrombophlebitis, and 1 saphenous nerve entrapment. The patient with saphenous nerve entrapment underwent immediate exploration, at which time the nerve was found to be entrapped by the sutures. If the patient has burning paresthesias in the distribution of the saphenous nerve immediately following surgery and these symptoms are made worse by knee extension, then immediate exploration is recommended. If there is only numbness in the saphenous nerve distribution, observation would be recommended. Exploration would be recommended if symptoms persisted after 6 to 12 weeks.

In conclusion, this study[99] has demonstrated that the location of the tear and the condition of the ACL are important factors in determining the success of meniscal repair. It is recommended that patients with concomitant medial meniscus and ACL tears undergo ACL reconstruction combined with meniscal repair. However, since there was a 62% healing rate in patients with an unrepaired ACL tear, consideration should still be given to meniscal repair in patients who refuse ACL reconstruction. Multiple permanent sutures should be used, and the patient must be counseled regarding the higher failure rate with this approach. Lateral meniscal repairs have a higher success rate and consideration should be given to lateral meniscus repair even in the presence of ACL insufficiency. The use of fibrin clot in isolated meniscal repair is currently recommended, especially for tears in the avascular inner two thirds of the meniscus. At HSS, MRI is used for the evaluation of meniscal healing, because it has been demonstrated to be as accurate as arthrography for this evaluation.[102]

ALL-INSIDE REPAIR TECHNIQUES

Suture Hook Technique

This technique[103] (Fig. 73) is limited to posterior horn tears amenable to repair with rim widths ≤ 2.5 mm. It significantly lessens the risk to posteri-

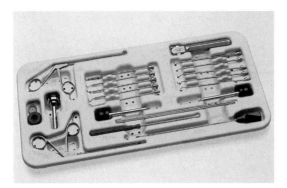

FIGURE 73
The suture hook set of instruments for all-inside meniscal repair. (Courtesy of Linvatec, Inc.)

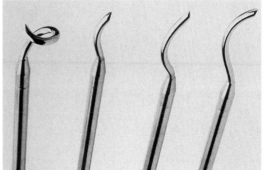

FIGURE 74
The suture hooks have different bends for use depending on the orientation of the meniscal tear. (Courtesy of Linvatec, Inc.)

or neurovascular structures, and is said to eliminate the complication of posterior capsular entrapment, although the latter may be of only theoretical concern. The posteromedial or posterolateral compartments must be well visualized by passing a 70° arthroscope through the intercondylar notch. The tear site is prepared by the previously described methods. A 7-mm cannula is placed through the posteromedial or posterolateral portal, and an appropriate suture hook is selected, usually the 45° angled one (Fig. 74). The preferred suture is a size 0 or #1 PDS, which is loaded in the suture hook. It is then introduced through the cannula, and a vertical suture is made starting through the rim and then the inner fragment. A probe introduced through an anterior portal may be needed to accomplish this. Once

the end of the suture hook is brought into view (Fig. 75), enough suture is advanced through it so that when the suture hook is withdrawn, there is abundant suture in the posterior joint space to be easily retrieved through the posterior cannula (Fig. 76). With both suture ends emerging through the posterior cannula, an arthroscopic knot tier is used to lay down slip knots alternated with half hitches with reversed direction of the throws and alternating posts (Fig. 77). Enough sutures are placed posteriorly to secure and coapt the tear site.

T-Fix Suture Anchor Technique

Another method of all-inside repair uses the T-Fix suture anchor device[104] (Smith and Nephew, Acufex Microsurgical Inc., Mansfield, MA)

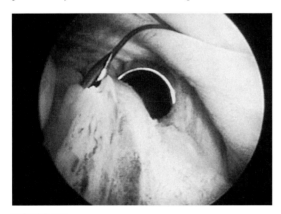

FIGURE 75
The suture hook instrument is used to place a vertical suture through the posterior horn of this left medial meniscal tear. (Courtesy of Linvatec, Inc.)

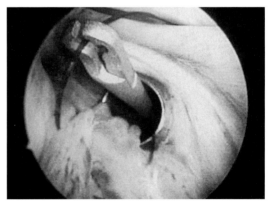

FIGURE 76
The suture shown in Figure 75 is being retrieved through the posteromedial cannula. (Courtesy of Linvatec, Inc.)

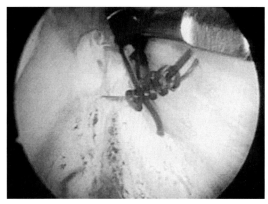

FIGURE 77
Arthroscopic knot tying has resulted in a secure suture. (Courtesy of Linvatec, Inc.)

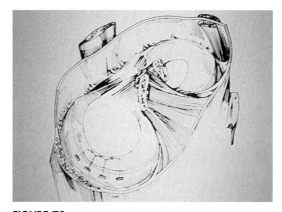

FIGURE 78
The deployment of 4 T-fix sutures for a tear of the medial meniscus. (Courtesy of Smith & Nephew, Inc.)

(Fig. 78). This technique uses a suture anchor consisting of a 3-mm polyacetal bar with a swedged on 2-0 nonabsorbable monofilament suture attached to it. The suture anchor is pre-loaded into a 17-gauge, 10-cm long spinal needle. This needle is coated with a protective coating of plastic. The needle has an obturator that pushes out and helps deploy the anchor in the meniscus or meniscal-capsular tissue once the needle is positioned appropriately across the tear site.

For both medial and lateral meniscal repairs, the arthroscope is placed in the contralateral portal and the needle comes in from the ipsilateral portal, thus providing a more radial orientation to the repair. For repairs of the central third of the meniscus, the needle is best introduced from the contralateral portal. Once a diagnostic sweep of the knee has been performed, and an appropriate meniscal tear identified, the tear site is rasped and prepared as has been previously described. A cannula is then placed through the ipsilateral portal, and a depth gauge is used to measure the distance across the tear site necessary for deployment of the anchor. It is recommended that 4 to 5 mm be added to this measurement to ensure adequate placement. The calculated figure is used to remove this amount of the protective plastic covering at the end of the needle (Fig. 79), thus insuring against overpenetration through the meniscus and into soft tissue beyond the capsule. The nee-

dle is then passed through the inner fragment of the meniscus, across the tear site, and into the peripheral portion of the meniscus (Fig. 80) until

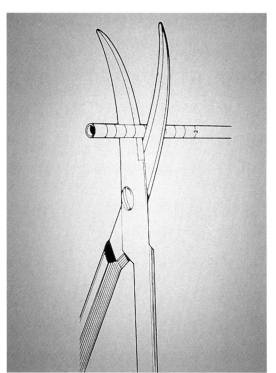

FIGURE 79
After measuring the distance across the tear site required for deployment of the T-fix device, 4 to 5 mm is added to this Figure and the protective plastic needle covering is cut accordingly. (Courtesy of Smith & Nephew, Inc.)

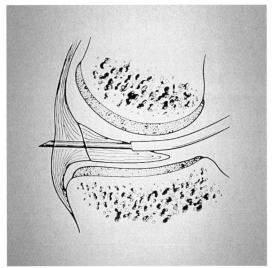

FIGURE 80
The needle is passed through the inner fragment of the meniscus, across the tear site and into the peripheral portion of the meniscus. (Courtesy of Smith & Nephew, Inc.)

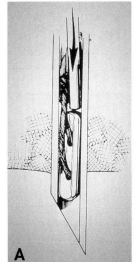
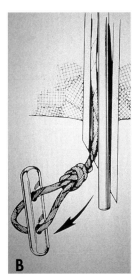

FIGURE 81
A, The obturator is about to push the polyacetal bar out of the end of the needle to deploy the bar. **B,** The bar is deployed. (Courtesy of Smith & Nephew, Inc.)

the cut end of the plastic sleeve abuts against the meniscus. A gentle give can be felt as the needle passes through the posterior meniscus. The obturator then pushes the polyacetal bar out of the end of the needle to deploy the bar within the peripheral aspect of the meniscus (Fig. 81). During this step, the surgeon should provide a gentle pull on the suture, thus assisting in the deployment of the bar, which should ideally be at a right angle to the needle. The stability of the device can be checked with this gentle pull. The needle and obturator are withdrawn from the joint, and a second T-fix anchor is placed approximately 3 to 4 mm away from the first on a horizontal plane (Fig. 82). After placement of the second anchor, the 2 suture ends are tied together using the T-fix knot pusher (Fig. 83). Four throws are usually adequate, but care must be taken to keep the first knot tight and secure before the third and fourth throws are made. For this reason, the first and second throws are identical so that the knot can be tightened. If the knot is loose, the meniscal fragment will not be tightly apposed to the rim fragment. The suture ends of the knot are then cut with arthroscopic scissors, keeping in mind that the knot will be sitting on top of the menis-

cus where, theoretically, there could be articular cartilage damage during flexion and extension of the knee postoperatively. After the completion of the first suture, additional ones are placed every 4 to 5 mm to provide secure fixation of the tear site (Fig. 78). The surgeon should try to place sutures alternating between superior and inferior surfaces of the meniscus.

Potential problems using this technique include the aforementioned potential abrasion from the knot, the difficulty in getting the first 2 knot throws tight, and difficulty providing fixation of a displaced bucket-handle tear of the meniscus. In the latter case, it has been suggested to initially place a mattress suture through the middle of the tear site in an inside-out method to hold the meniscus reduced while the T-fix anchors are placed. At the end of the procedure, the holding suture can be removed so that a posterior incision does not have to be made. Also, it is accepted in the literature that horizontally placed sutures are weaker than vertical sutures, and the latter are difficult to place using this technique.

Barrett and associates[105] in 1996 reported on their results using the T-fix device. They had used it in 62 patients, 46 T-fix alone, 10 hybrid cases,

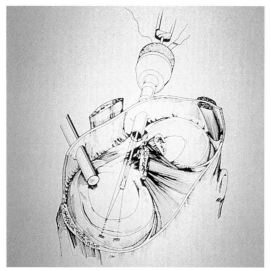

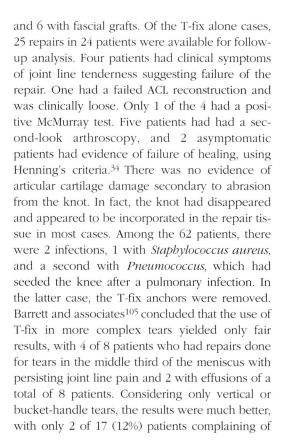

FIGURE 82
Two adjacent sutures are tied together by means of an arthroscopic knot tyer, thus producing a horizontal mattress suture. (Courtesy of Smith & Nephew, Inc.)

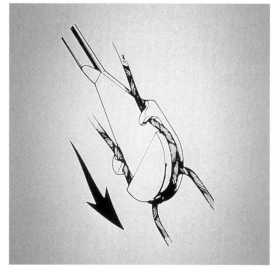

FIGURE 83
An arthroscopic knot is tied using the special knot pusher. (Courtesy of Smith & Nephew, Inc.)

and 6 with fascial grafts. Of the T-fix alone cases, 25 repairs in 24 patients were available for follow-up analysis. Four patients had clinical symptoms of joint line tenderness suggesting failure of the repair. One had a failed ACL reconstruction and was clinically loose. Only 1 of the 4 had a positive McMurray test. Five patients had had a second-look arthroscopy, and 2 asymptomatic patients had evidence of failure of healing, using Henning's criteria.[34] There was no evidence of articular cartilage damage secondary to abrasion from the knot. In fact, the knot had disappeared and appeared to be incorporated in the repair tissue in most cases. Among the 62 patients, there were 2 infections, 1 with *Staphylococcus aureus,* and a second with *Pneumococcus,* which had seeded the knee after a pulmonary infection. In the latter case, the T-fix anchors were removed. Barrett and associates[105] concluded that the use of T-fix in more complex tears yielded only fair results, with 4 of 8 patients who had repairs done for tears in the middle third of the meniscus with persisting joint line pain and 2 with effusions of a total of 8 patients. Considering only vertical or bucket-handle tears, the results were much better, with only 2 of 17 (12%) patients complaining of

persisting joint line tenderness. There was no evidence of an adverse reaction secondary to a permanent foreign body in the knee joint in any of their patients.

Meniscus Arrow

Albrecht-Olsen and associates[106] in 1993 were the first to report on a polylactic acid biodegradable arrow for use in the fixation of bucket-handle tears. The goal of this all-inside technique was to eliminate the need for a posterior incision, reducing the risk of neurovascular injury, and to simplify the fixation procedure.

Meniscus arrows,[106] approved by the FDA in 1997, are available in 10-, 13-, and 16-mm lengths (Fig. 84). Arrows may remain in the joint for over 1 year before they disappear by hydrolysis. This constitutes a benign process and does not evoke an inflammatory reaction.

Pullout Strength of Arrows Albrecht-Olsen and associates[107] also reported on the pullout strength of meniscus arrows compared to horizontally placed 2-0 Ethibond sutures in bovine menisci. They found that there was no significant difference between the arrows and the sutures, the

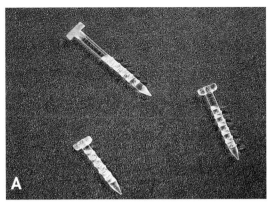
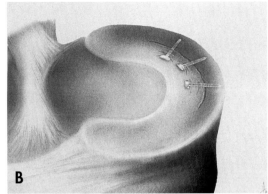

FIGURE 84
A, Meniscus arrows come in 3 lengths: 10, 13, and 16 mm. **B,** Artist's depiction of 3 meniscus arrows placed in the meniscus. (Courtesy of Bionx, Inc.)

strength of the arrows being 53 N and that of the sutures 49 N. One criticism of their study is that they did not compare the arrows to vertically oriented sutures, which are theoretically stronger and more commonly used than horizontal sutures.

Dervin and associates[108] studied the pullout strength of the arrow compared to vertically oriented 2-0 Ethibond sutures in human cadaver menisci. They found the mean failure load for the suture group was 58.3 N compared with 29.6 N for the arrow group ($p < 0.001$). All sutures failed by rupture at the knot but did not pull through the meniscus. All but 1 of the arrows failed by pulling out of the meniscus. The arrows also permitted gapping at the repair site at considerably lesser loads than the sutures.

Boenisch and associates[109] performed a pullout study in young bovine lateral menisci comparing arrows of different lengths to 2-0 Ty-cron sutures (American Cyanamid Co., Danbury, CT) placed both horizontally and vertically. Comparing the horizontally versus vertically placed sutures, they found breakage strengths of 68 N and 72 N, respectively. The sutures broke at the knots. They found that the vertically oriented sutures had a significantly higher stiffness compared to the horizontally placed sutures. In the arrow study, they found the number of barbs traversing the tear site, starting 5 mm to the inner side of the tear, to be 3 for 10-mm arrows, 7 to 8 for 13-mm arrows, and

10 for 16-mm arrows. Because the strength of the fixation depends on the number of barbs engaged in the rim side, their results showed a pullout strength of only 18 N with the 10-mm arrows, 39 N with the 13-mm arrows, and 53 N using the 16-mm arrows. If the distance from the tear site was reduced to 2 mm, then the strength of the 10-mm arrows increased to 35 N. In all cases, the pullout strength of the arrows was significantly weaker than that of the sutures. However, even with a lower figure for pullout, the arrows still probably have adequate strength to maintain meniscal tear coaptation during the healing phase.

Meniscus Arrow Surgical Technique After a diagnostic arthroscopy has been performed and a reparable meniscus tear identified in the red-red or red-white zones, tear site preparation is done as described in the previous techniques. If the meniscus tear is being repaired in conjunction with an ACL reconstruction, the meniscus should be repaired first.

The instrumentation consists of a straight cannula, a pair of right and left curved cannulas, and a pair of up and down curved cannulas (Fig. 85). Only the straight cannula, the most commonly used of the 5, has an additional small lumen and channel for passage of a stabilizing pin into the meniscus so that the cannula is less likely to slip once placed against the substance of the meniscus (Fig. 86). Select the proper cannula to allow

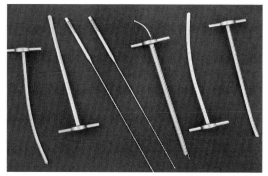

FIGURE 85

Meniscus arrow instrumentation, including a variety of cannulas, a trochar, and an obturator. (Courtesy of Bionx, Inc.)

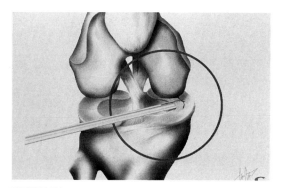

FIGURE 86

A stabilizing pin is driven into the meniscus through a small piggybacked sleeve. Only the straight cannula comes with the extra sleeve. (Courtesy of Bionx, Inc.)

as perpendicular an approach to the tear as possible. The cannulas were created with curves to minimize the possibility of needing an additional portal for arrow implantation.

For tears of the posterior horn of either the medial or lateral meniscus, arrow lengths should be either 13 or 16 mm, and arrows should be inserted from an ipsilateral portal. However, caution should be used when using 16-mm long arrows in small knees with more peripheral tears to reduce the risk of posterolateral neurovascular injury, or an irritable arrow point. For tears of the

middle third of the medial or lateral meniscus, arrow lengths should be 10 or 13 mm, and arrows should be introduced from a contralateral portal. For the rare tears of the anterior horn, 10-mm arrows should be inserted from the opposite mid-patella medial or lateral portal (Fig. 87).

Insert the selected cannula with the obturator in place to avoid snagging soft tissue anteriorly on insertion. Remove the obturator, grip the meniscus using the sharp tip of the cannula, and effect any additional reduction of the tear that may need to be done. The cannula should be

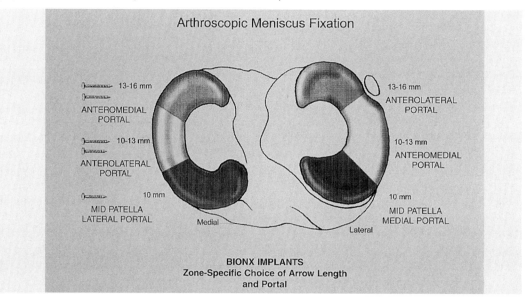

FIGURE 87

The length of the arrow and the portal of entry depend on the tear location. (Courtesy of Bionx, Inc.)

placed on the superior surface of the meniscus so that there is at least 3 mm of meniscus substance on the mobile inner fragment to allow for placement of the T-head of the arrow. It is very difficult to place arrows on the inferior surface of the meniscus, and adequate fixation can be obtained by arrows placed through the superior surface of the meniscus only. It is extremely important for the surgeon to maintain the cannula position throughout the arrow placement by pressing the heel of his or her hand against the knee and firmly grasping the cannula. For posterior tears, place the first arrow in the most posterior position and then move to the center of the tear with the second arrow. Place all other arrows by alternating posterior and anterior to the center arrow. For all other tears, place the center arrow first, then alternate anteriorly and posteriorly to the center arrow. To maximize fixation, keep the cannula and the T-head of the arrow as parallel as possible to the joint line and meniscus.

While maintaining firm pressure on the cannula, insert the cutting needle into the cannula and the meniscus; it should be seated against the head of the cannula when fully inserted (Fig. 88). The needle protrudes 13 mm from the end of the cannula and can be used as a gauge for the selection of the proper length arrow. Remove the needle and shut off the irrigation when inserting an arrow, otherwise there is a risk of the arrow being propelled out of the cannula and onto the floor by the force of the pressurized intra-articular fluid. To avoid potential postoperative pain or injury to posterior structures, the arrows should not protrude more than 1 mm into the capsule. The appropriate arrow is inserted into the cannula and pushed down it with the blunt obturator. The irrigation flow can be restarted. Drive the arrow into the meniscus by gently tapping with a mallet (Fig. 89). The obturator must seat fully against the cannula to assure that the T-head of the arrow has been fully countersunk (Fig. 90). If the T-head can be palpated with a probe, then the cannula should be placed back over the arrow and tapped again. Maintaining the cannula perpendicular to the tear and meniscus, shift the cannula to a new position or insert a different cannula to insert the next arrow, maintaining 5 mm between the arrow shafts (not the T-heads) (Fig. 90).

There is a new meniscus arrow inserter that allows the surgeon to load up to 4 arrows into a magazine that is loaded into a gun. The arrow is inserted by pulling a trigger and firing the gun (Fig. 91).

Advantages of the use of meniscus arrows are ease of use, avoidance of posterior incisions for needle retrieval, and speed of the technique. Arrow disadvantages include the high cost of the arrow, the difficulty of introducing arrows on the inferior surface of the meniscus, lower pullout

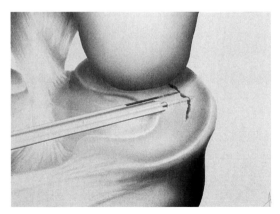

FIGURE 88
Once the inner meniscal fragment has been reduced and stabilized, a 13-mm trochar is pushed across the tear, preparing a channel for the arrow. (Courtesy of Bionx, Inc.)

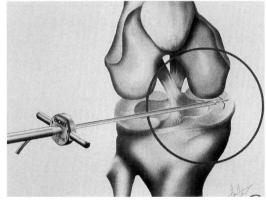

FIGURE 89
The appropriately sized arrow has been tapped across the tear site. (Courtesy of Bionx, Inc.)

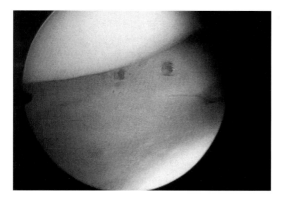

FIGURE 90
This unstable vertical longitudinal tear of the posterior horn of the left medial meniscus has been fixed with 2 arrows placed approximately 5 mm apart on the superior surface. (Reproduced with permission of Primal Pictures, London, England)

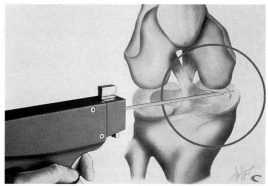

FIGURE 91
The meniscus arrow gun can be preloaded with up to four arrows, which are fired across the meniscus without making a preliminary pilot hole. (Courtesy of Bionx, Inc.)

strength versus vertically oriented sutures, difficulty inserting fibrin clot in isolated meniscus repair cases, and the potential of articular cartilage abrasion if the arrow is left too high on the superior surface of the meniscus. Arrows also can be inserted too deeply into partially degenerative menisci, thus losing their holding strength. Cannon prefers a hybrid technique using meniscus arrows for the posterior horn tears amenable for this technique, and then using sutures if the

tear extends into the midcentral portion of the meniscus. Similar to other meniscus repair techniques, the arrow cannot be used for all types of meniscus tears. The surgeon must have in his or her armamentarium more than 1 meniscus repair instrumentation.

Because of the newness of the technique, aside from the Danish study mentioned above, there are no long-term results to report. In a survey in February 1998, 296 cases using meniscus

TABLE 1

THE AGE DISTRIBUTION IN THE MENISCUS ARROW SURVEY

Age (Yrs)	No.
10 to 19	94
20 to 29	95
30 to 39	60
40 to 49	31
50 to 59	8
60 to 69	1
70 to 79	1

TABLE 2

THE TEAR LENGTH DISTRIBUTION IN THE MENISCUS ARROW SURVEY

Tear Length (mm)	No.
0 to 10	66
11 to 20	78
21 to 30	62
31 to 40	38
41 to 50	17
51 to 60	2

arrows were collected. The number of arrows averaged 1.5 per meniscus repair, indicating that most surgeons are using the arrow along with sutures in a hybrid manner. Tables 1 and 2 show the age distribution and tear lengths in this study. The tear patterns were predominantly of 2 types, vertical longitudinal (186), and bucket-handle (78). There were 86 arrows placed in red-red tears, 146 arrows placed in red-white tears, and 27 arrows placed in white-white tears. Only 17 arrows were reportedly placed through the inferior surface of the meniscus. Complications included 4 infections, 3 loose extruded arrows, and 1 each of pain over the arrow tip, reflex sympathetic dystrophy, a stiff knee, and deep venous thrombosis. Eighteen reoperations were performed. In 4 instances, there were fragmented arrows still in situ; 2 arrows were found loose, but still in place; and 4 cases in which arrows or arrow parts were removed.

Another new biodegradable technique reported by Koukoubis and associates[110] uses an absorbable staple. It consists of 2 rigid barbed legs, made of a copolymer of polyglycolic acid and polylactic acid, connected by a flexible suture made of the same absorbable material (Fig. 92). In a canine study comparing it to 3-0 PDS suture, absorption of the staple began by 3 months and was almost complete by 1 year. Mechanically, the staple provided greater tensile strength augmentation of the meniscus than suture fixation for up

to 4 months. In the long-term, there was no difference in healing rates between the staple and suture. Several companies are actively pursuing the development of other biodegradable devices for meniscus fixation (Fig. 93).

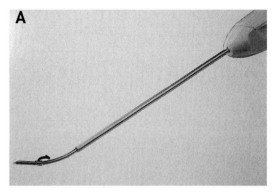

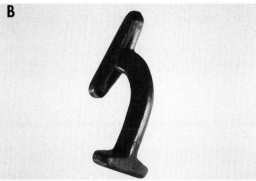

FIGURE 93
A, This all-inside technique uses an inserter and a biodegradable tack **(B)**. (Courtesy of Mitek, Inc.)

Complications of All-Inside Repair

Because of the relative newness of these techniques, little has been written on this subject. General complications exist for these procedures as they do for other techniques. Broken instrumentation may occur. T-fix anchors are not biodegradable and have the potential of causing chronic irritation. Arrows, although biodegradable, remain in the joint relatively intact for up to a year, and may break and become loose bodies. They can be inserted too deep, and cause irritation either of posterior structures, or irritate the skin if the arrows are too long in the midcentral region of the meniscus (Fig. 94).

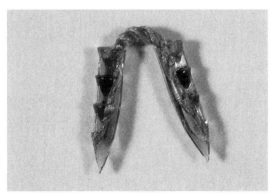

FIGURE 92
A new alternative all-inside technique uses gun that fires a barbed staple across the meniscus. A close-up of the barbed staple is shown. (Courtesy of Surgical Dynamics.)

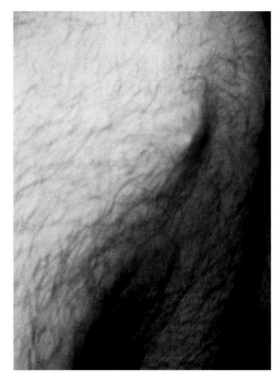

FIGURE 94

This patient was experiencing sharp, darting pain from the points of two 13-mm meniscus arrows that had been inserted too deeply into a tear of the middle third of the medial meniscus of this right knee.

DISCUSSION

Comparing results of meniscus repair in the literature is quite difficult because of the variety of techniques used (open; arthroscopic outside-in, inside-out, and all-inside) and the variables within each series (patient age, chronicity and type of tear, rim width, concomitant procedures, medial versus lateral, and more). Further clouding the issue is the definition of a successful meniscus repair. Clinical results overestimate the number of anatomic successes, as has been illustrated in a number of second-look studies.[34,81,91] The best method of objective follow-up in order to assess the outcome following meniscus repair is second-look arthroscopy, but with the advent of managed care, it is difficult to justify to an insurance carrier the need for a second-look arthroscopy.

Magnetic resonance imaging (MRI) studies[111,112] have shown that in the majority of menis-cus repairs, there was universal persistence of a grade 3 signal suggestive of a complete tear at follow-up. In a goat model, Ritchie and associates[113] showed a false positive rate of 67% using MRI for assessing the results of meniscus repair. In contrast, a recent study[102] showed that using newer imaging techniques, MRI was as accurate as conventional arthrography in assessing the state of healing of repaired menisci.

Rim width is considered the most important predictive factor for healing, because tears approaching the meniscocapsular junction (0 to 3 mm) have the greatest capacity for healing.[34] Tenuta and Arciera[114] found that no meniscal repair with a rim width greater than 4 mm healed. However, Rubman and associates[115] found that 159 of 198 tears that extended into the avascular zone had successful repairs. Only 20% required further surgery for symptoms consistent with a possible meniscal tear.

As has been reported previously in this monograph, Cannon, Rosenberg, and Rodeo found that repairs of the lateral meniscus generally have a higher success rate than those of the medial meniscus,[34,37,81,89,90] but Horibe and associates[116] found the opposite to be true. Most authors report no significant difference in healing rates of acute versus chronic tears.[81,116] Eggli and associates[76] and Henning and associates,[83] however, found improved healing rates in meniscal repairs done within 8 weeks of injury. Also, age does not appear to have a detrimental influence on healing.[91,116] After Cannon and Vittori[91] reported that meniscus repair associated with ACL reconstruction heals statistically significantly better than meniscus repair done in ACL-stable knees, multiple authors have substantiated this observation.[34,114,117] After ACL reconstruction is carried out, there is less stress on the repair site because the tibia no longer subluxes anteriorly. Thomas Tiling (personal communication, April 1991, Kyoto, Japan) found that biopsies of isolated meniscal tears showed degenerative changes present, whereas biopsies of meniscal tears associated with ACL tears revealed normal meniscal tissue.

Except under unusual circumstances, meniscus repair alone in an ACL-deficient patient is not recommended. Jensen and associates[118] reported 7 of 10 failures in patients with nonsurgical treatment of ACL tears. DeHaven and associates[90] had a 38% retear rate in repairs done in ACL-deficient patients. Kimura and associates[119] found a statistically significant reduced healing rate ($p < 0.005$) in ACL-deficient patients. Miller and associates,[120] in a goat study, found a significantly reduced healing rate of repairs done when the ACL was sectioned.

In contrast to Cannon's results, which showed that patients with a history of locking had a statistically significant decreased healing rate compared to patients without a history of locking, Scott and associates[34] did not find any difference in healing rates.

Further work has to be done before the use of fibrin clot as an adjunct in the repair technique can be strongly recommended. Cannon (Fig. 57) showed that the use of fibrin clot improved the healing rate in isolated meniscal repairs ($p = 0.10$), and Henning and associates[82] reported improved healing rates using clot for isolated repairs, but in a goat study, Port and associates[121] showed no statistically significant advantage in the use of fibrin clot compared to sutures alone.

There are not many long-term reports of the outcome of meniscus repair, and the reported results vary considerably. Morgan and Casscells[33] reported a 98.6% overall clinical success rate, whereas Cannon and Morgan[81] reported only 48% healed and incompletely healed menisci in 25 isolated repairs in ACL-stable knees. DeHaven and associates,[122] reporting on an average 10.9-year follow-up of 33 open meniscal repairs, noted that the average time between surgery and clinical evidence of failure was 4 years. There was a 79% survival rate of repaired menisci. Scott and associates[34] reported only a 3% reoperation rate for 240 patients who had had meniscal repair. It is likely that the percentage of successfully healed meniscal repairs will steadily drop off with the passage of time, and that the early assessment of healing by second-look arthroscopy or arthrogram recommended by Henning gives a best case scenario.

How long do menisci stay healed? Certainly there are patients who initially are asymptomatic and later become symptomatic, complaining of 1

or more symptoms of joint line pain, clicking, locking, or swelling. These patients may never have healed, based on anatomic assessment. For example, an 18-year-old male who presented with a displaced bucket-handle tear of his medial meniscus underwent repair using 6 sutures but no fibrin clot in January 1987. An arthrogram 5 months later revealed that the repair had failed. The patient was advised not to engage in any contact sports and remained asymptomatic for 31 months until he redisplaced his meniscus when bending down to pick up an object from the floor. The patient wanted to have re-repair done, and this was accomplished using 8 sutures and fibrin clot. An arthrogram 16 months later revealed the meniscus to be completely healed. He twisted his knee again 4 years after his second surgery, and on his own, obtained another arthrogram, which again revealed the repair to be completely healed.

As patients with meniscal repair are followed up for longer periods of time, there will be increasing numbers of failures. This will present a challenge to the orthopaedic surgeon as to whether to urge the patient with a failed repair to undergo re-repair with its obligatory lengthy rehabilitation. Re-repair of failed meniscal tears certainly should be considered in individual cases. Some patients, especially athletes, will outright reject the suggestion of re-repair because of the lengthy rehabilitation involved, and opt for a quick partial meniscectomy in order to get on with their sports or life activities. Other patients understand the long-term importance of the meniscus, and want to proceed with re-repair even though the chances of a successful outcome are considerably lower than with a primary repair. Cannon (unpublished data) has had experience with 16 cases of re-repair. Eight of them were anatomically assessed, and 50% of them had successfully healed. Most menisci undergoing re-repair had evidence of degenerative changes. As an example, a 40-year-old woman presented with a retear of a medial meniscal repair done in conjunction with an ACL reconstruction by Cannon 13 years previously. She had had an arthroscopic second look done 4 years after her initial repair, and the repair looked completely healed. A posteroanterior bent knee standing radiograph revealed only slight joint space narrowing, supporting the protective effect that her first meniscus repair had in protecting her joint from significant degenerative arthritis. At the time of her re-repair, the meniscus was moderately degenerative, but torn in the same location as the original tear. The re-repair was done with multiple nonabsorbable sutures using the Henning technique. Her follow-up is too short to state whether this re-repair will hold up with time.

There are many different recommended rehabilitation techniques reported in the literature. Some recommend immediate full weightbearing and a full range of motion, whereas others recommend full weightbearing but keep the knee in an extended position. Others keep the patient nonweightbearing for up to 6 weeks with or without restricted range of motion. The final answer is not known, and almost any protocol that the surgeon wishes to follow is probably reasonable. Arnoczky has shown that the least amount of motion of the menisci occurs between 15° and 60° of flexion, as discussed earlier in this monograph. He would recommend keeping the knee within this range of motion until early healing has occurred. Dowdy and associates,[71] in a canine study, showed that motion benefitted meniscal healing by preventing a significant decrease in collagen production which occurred if immobilization was continued for 10 weeks. Klein and associates,[123] in another canine study, showed significant meniscal atrophy with immobilization. Djurasovic and associates[85] reported a significant reduction in aggrecan synthesis in the meniscus in immobilized knees.

Important points to consider in designing a rehabilitation protocol are that immobilization, in addition to the detrimental points mentioned above, can produce arthrofibrosis when meniscal repair is combined with ACL reconstruction. Austin and Sherman[93] reported a 10% incidence of arthrofibrosis when meniscal repair was performed with ACL reconstruction, whereas only a 6% incidence when performed in an ACL-deficient, nonreconstructed knee. Therefore, with this combination of procedures, early motion is justified. In order to lessen the incidence of flexion contractures after meniscus repair of displaced bucket-handle tears done in conjunction with ACL reconstruction, Shelbourne and Johnson[124] recommended staging the surgeries, performing the meniscus repair first, allowing the patient to regain range of motion before readmitting the patient for the ACL reconstruction.

Barber[125] favored an unrestricted rehabilitation protocol. In his study, 1 group of patients was braced and kept nonweightbearing for 6 weeks, with no pivoting sports for 6 months. In a second group, he allowed full, unbraced motion with immediate unlimited weightbearing and unrestricted return to pivoting sports once they had no effusion, full extension and at least 120° of flexion. All repairs were performed in an inside-out technique. In the restricted group of 58 repairs, the failure rate was 19%. In the unrestricted group of 40 repairs, the failure rate was only 10%. These results would favor an unrestricted protocol. In a subsequent report, Barber and Click[117] concluded that there was no need to modify the rehabilitation program for meniscal repairs performed in conjunction with ACL reconstruction. Buseck and Noyes[126] reached the same conclusion.

Return to sports is also a controversial point. The conservative viewpoint would be to prevent patients from returning to sports until 6 months postoperatively. Roeddecker and associates' work[64] showing that repaired canine menisci took 6 months to regain 62% strength would justify this position.

Shelbourne and associates[127] allowed patients with meniscal repair to follow a rehabilitation program that allowed immediate range of motion and weightbearing as tolerated. They allowed patients to return to activities and sports at their own pace without significantly altering the outcome of repair. More investigative studies need to be done to arrive at the ideal postoperative rehabilitative program.

FUTURE DIRECTIONS
There will be further development of barbs, tacks, and arrows to make meniscus repair more easily

accomplished using an all-inside technique with the avoidance of posterior incisions. Techniques that are faster will be attractive to more surgeons, prompting them to repair tears that previously were excised. But surgeons should not endorse techniques just because they are fast. Ochi and associates[128] in an organ culture model, showed that free autogenous synovial tissue grafts in meniscal defects were superior to fibrin glue. Applying this finding clinically would make for a technically demanding procedure, but Kimura and associates[119] reported 7 out of 7 meniscal repairs in the avascular zone healed when they implanted a vascularized synovial pedicle into the tear site.

Challenges for future research include the further development of biodegradable fixation devices, research into whether specific growth factors will enhance meniscal healing, the development of carriers for these growth factors, the use of collagen scaffolds to replace segments of the meniscus,[129,130] and scientific studies on the fate of meniscal allograft transplants.[131]

Robert Jackson is working on a new and exciting concept for repair. Preliminary work on meniscus repair in rabbits and sheep using photodynamic tissue welding with 1,8 naphthalimide dye and blue laser light are promising. The possibility of healing meniscus tears by covalently bonding collagen molecules is extremely exciting. Tears in the avascular zone could be bonded together. There would be less morbidity and avoidance of foreign material implanted in menisci.

SUMMARY

In the last decade, arthroscopic meniscus repair has become established as the treatment of choice for many meniscal lesions previously managed by meniscectomy. Anatomic and clinical evidence supports meniscus repair for reparable tears, especially in adolescents and young adults undergoing ACL reconstruction, whereas partial meniscectomy is appropriate for older patients. In patients with ACL-deficient knees, the surgeon should broaden the criteria for repair compared to isolated meniscal repair in ACL-stable patients because of the increased successful outcomes in this group. Meniscal repair, especially of the medial meniscus, is a key in providing optimal long-term stability when performing ACL reconstruction.

Meniscus repair is a demanding technique that requires the skill of an experienced arthroscopist. Special suturing tools and techniques are often required, but these are no substitute for appropriate selection and thorough preparation of specific tears that are likely to heal. The use of new biodegradable barbs, tacks, and arrows will make the technique of meniscal repair faster and easier to accomplish, and hence more surgeons are likely to perform them.

REFERENCES

1. Annandale T: An operation for displaced semilunar cartilage. *Br Med J* 1885;1:779.

2. Bland-Sutton J (ed): *Ligaments, Their Nature and Morphology,* ed 2. London, England, HK Lewis, 1897.

3. King D: The healing of semilunar cartilages. *J Bone Joint Surg* 1936;18:333–342.

4. King D: The function of semilunar cartilages. *J Bone Joint Surg* 1936;18:1069–1076.

5. Fairbank TJ: Knee joint changes after meniscectomy. *J Bone Joint Surg* 1948;30B:664–670.

6. Huckell JR: Is meniscectomy a benign procedure? A long-term follow-up study. *Can J Surg* 1965;8:254–260.

7. Gear MW: The late results of meniscectomy. *Br J Surg* 1967;54:270–272.

8. Jackson JP: Degenerative changes in the knee after meniscectomy. *Br Med J* 1968;2:525–527.

9. Tapper EM, Hoover NW: Late results after meniscectomy. *J Bone Joint Surg* 1969;51A:517–526.

10. Appel H: Late results after meniscectomy in the knee joint: A clinical and roentgenologic follow-up investigation. *Acta Orthop Scand* 1970;133(Suppl):1–111.

11. Johnson RJ, Kettelkamp DB, Clark W, Leaverton P, et al: Factors effecting late results after meniscectomy. *J Bone Joint Surg* 1974;56A:719–729.

12. Krause WR, Pope MH, Johnson RJ, Wilder DG: Mechanical changes in the knee after meniscectomy. *J Bone Joint Surg* 1976;58A:599–604.

13. Cox JS, Cordell LD: The degenerative effects of medial meniscus tears in dogs' knees. *Clin Orthop* 1977;125:236–242.

14. Hargreaves DJ, Seedhom BB: Abstract: On the "bucket handle" tear: Partial or total meniscectomy? A quantitative study. *J Bone Joint Surg* 1979;61B:381.

15. Northmore-Ball MD, Dandy DJ: Long-term results of arthroscopic partial meniscectomy. *Clin Orthop* 1982;167:34–42.

16. Lynch MA, Henning CE, Glick KR Jr: Knee joint surface changes: Long-term follow-up meniscus tear treatment in stable anterior cruciate ligament reconstructions. *Clin Orthop* 1983;172:148–153.

17. Allen PR, Denham RA, Swan AV: Late degenerative changes after meniscectomy: Factors affecting the knee after operation. *J Bone Joint Surg* 1984;66B:666–671.

18. Veth RP: Clinical significance of knee joint changes after meniscectomy. *Clin Orthop* 1985;198:56–60.

19. O'Brien WR, Warren RF, Friederich NF, et al: Degenerative arthritis of the knee following anterior cruciate ligament injury: A multi-center, long-term follow-up study. *Orthop Trans* 1989;13:546.

20. Sommerlath KG: Results of meniscal repair and partial meniscectomy in stable knees. *Int Orthop* 1991;15:347–350.

21. Burks RT, Metcalf MH, Metcalf RW: Fifteen-year follow-up of arthroscopic partial meniscectomy. *Arthroscopy* 1997;13:673–679.

22. Ikeuchi H: Surgery under arthroscopic control, in Proceedings of the Societe Internationale d'Arthroscopie. *Rheumatology* 1975;57–62.

23. DeHaven KE: Peripheral meniscus repair: An alternative to meniscectomy. *Orthop Trans* 1981;5:399–400.

24. Price CT, Allen WC: Ligament repair in the knee with preservation of the meniscus. *J Bone Joint Surg* 1978;60A:61–65.

25. Cassidy RE, Shaffer AJ: Repair of peripheral meniscus tears: A preliminary report. *Am J Sports Med* 1981;9:209–214.

26. Dolan WA, Bhaskar G: Peripheral meniscus repair: A clinical pathological study of 75 cases. *Orthop Trans* 1983;7:503–504.

27. Hamberg P, Gillquist J, Lysholm J: Suture of new and old peripheral meniscus tears. *J Bone Joint Surg* 1983;65A:193–197.

28. Henning CE: Arthroscopic repair of meniscus tears. *Orthopedics* 1983;6:1130–1132.

29. Clancy WG Jr, Graf BK: Arthroscopic meniscal repair. *Orthopedics* 1983;6:1125–1129.

30. Warren RF: Arthroscopic meniscus repair. *Arthroscopy* 1985;1:170–172.

31. Rosenberg T, Scott S, Paulos L: Arthroscopic surgery: Repair of peripheral detachment of the meniscus. *Contemp Orthop* 1985;10:43–50.

32. Barber FA, Stone RG: Meniscal repair: An arthroscopic technique. *J Bone Joint Surg* 1985;67B:39–41.

33. Morgan CD, Casscells SW: Arthroscopic meniscus repair: A safe approach to the posterior horns. *Arthroscopy* 1986;2:3–12.

34. Scott GA, Jolly BL, Henning CE: Combined posterior incision and arthroscopic intra-articular repair of the meniscus: An examination of factors affecting healing. *J Bone Joint Surg* 1986;68A:847–861.

35. DeHaven KE, Black KP, Griffiths HS: Meniscus repair. *Orthop Trans* 1987;11:469.

36. Barber FA: Meniscus repair: Results of an arthroscopic technique. *Arthroscopy* 1987;3:25–30.

37. Jakob RP, Staubli HU, Zuber K, Esser M: The arthroscopic meniscal repair: Techniques and clinical experience. *Am J Sports Med* 1988;16:137–142.

38. Arnoczky SP, Warren RF, Spivak JM: Meniscal repair using an exogenous fibrin clot: An experimental study in dogs. *J Bone Joint Surg* 1988;70A:1209–1217.

39. Warren R, Arnoczky SP, Wickiewicz TL: Anatomy of the knee, in Nicholas JA, Hershman EB (eds): *The Lower Extremity and Spine in Sports Medicine*. St. Louis, MO, CV Mosby, 1986, pp 657–694.

40. Ghadially FN (ed): *Fine Structure of Synovial Joints: A Text and Atlas of the Ultrastructure of Normal and Pathological Articular Tissues*. London, England, Butterworth, 1983, pp 103–144.

41. Ghadially FN, Thomas I, Yong N, Lalonde JM: Ultrastructure of rabbit semilunar cartilages. *J Anat* 1978;125:499–517.

42. McDevitt CA, Webber RJ: The ultrastructure and biochemistry of meniscal cartilage. *Clin Orthop* 1990;252:8–18.

43. Eyre DR, Koob TJ, Chun LE: Biochemistry of the meniscus: Unique profile of collagen types and site-dependent variations in composition. *Orthop Trans* 1983;7:264.

44. Bullough PG, Munuera L, Murphy J, Weinstein AM: The strength of the menisci of the knee as it relates to their fine structure. *J Bone Joint Surg* 1970;52B:564–567.

45. Yasui K: Three dimensional architecture of human normal menisci. *J Japan Orthop Assoc* 1978;52:391–399.

46. Aspden RM, Yarker YE, Hukins DW: Collagen orientations in the meniscus of the knee joint. *J Anat* 1985;140:371–380.

47. Adams ME, Billingham ME, Muir H: The glycosaminoglycans in menisci in experimental and natural osteoarthritis. *Arthritis Rheum* 1983;26:69–76.

48. Ingman AM, Ghosh P, Taylor TK: Variation of collagenous and non-collagenous proteins of human knee joint menisci with age and degeneration. *Gerontology* 1974;20:212–223.

49. Nakano T, Thompson JR, Aherne FX: Distribution of glycosaminoglycans and the non-reducible collagen crosslink, pyridinoline in porcine menisci. *Can J Vet Res* 1986;50:532–536.

50. Herwig J, Egner E, Buddecke E: Chemical changes of human knee joint menisci in various stages of degeneration. *Ann Rheum Dis* 1984;43:635–640.

51. McNicol D, Roughley PJ: Extraction and characterization of proteoglycan from human meniscus. *Biochem J* 1980:185:705–713.

52. Roughley PJ, McNicol D, Santer V, Buckwalter J: The presence of a cartilage-like proteoglycan in the adult human meniscus. *Biochem J* 1981;197:77–83.

53. Fife RS: Identification of link proteins and a 116,000-Dalton matrix protein in canine meniscus. *Arch Biochem Biophys* 1985;240:682–688.

54. Miller RR, McDevitt CA: Thrombospondin in ligament, meniscus and intervertebral disc. *Biochim Biophys Acta* 1991;1115:85–88.

55. Ahmed AM, Burke DL: In-vitro measurement of static pressure distribution in synovial joints: Part I. Tibial surface of the knee. *J Biomech Eng* 1983;105:216–225.

56. Baratz ME, Fu FH, Mengato R: Meniscal tears: The effect of meniscectomy and of repair on intraarticular contact areas and stress in the human knee. A preliminary report. *Am J Sports Med* 1986;14:270–275.

57. Seedhom BB, Hargreaves DJ: Transmission of the load in the knee joint with special reference to the role of the menisci: Part II. Experimental results, discussion and conclusions. *Eng Med* 1979;8:220–228.

58. Voloshin AS, Wosk J: Shock absorption of meniscectomized and painful knees: A comparative in vivo study. *J Biomed Eng* 1983;5:157-161.

59. Radin EL, Rose RM: Role of subchondral bone in the initiation and progression of cartilage damage. *Clin Orthop* 1986;213:34–40.

60. Levy IM, Torzilli PA, Warren RF: The effect of medial meniscectomy on anterior-posterior motion of the knee. *J Bone Joint Surg* 1982;64A:883–888.

61. Levy IM, Torzilli PA, Gould JD, Warren RF: The effect of lateral meniscectomy on motion of the knee. *J Bone Joint Surg* 1989;71A:401–406.

62. Arnoczky SP, Warren RF: Microvasculature of the human meniscus. *Am J Sports Med* 1982;10:90–95.

63. Arnoczky SP, Warren RF: The microvasculature of the meniscus and its response to injury: An experimental study in the dog. *Am J Sports Med* 1983;11:131–141.

64. Roeddecker K, Muennich U, Nagelschmidt M: Meniscal healing: A biomechanical study. *J Surg Res* 1994;56:20–27.

65. Henning CE, Lynch MA, Clark JR: Vascularity for healing of meniscus repairs. *Arthroscopy* 1987;3:13–18.

66. Veth RP, den Heeten GJ, Jansen HW, Nielsen HK: Repair of the meniscus: An experimental investigation in rabbits. *Clin Orthop* 1983;175:258–262.

67. Webber RJ, Harris MG, Hough AJ Jr: Cell culture of rabbit meniscal fibrochondrocytes: Proliferative and synthetic response to growth factors and ascorbate. *J Orthop Res* 1985;3:36–42.

68. Webber RJ, York L, Vander Schilden JL, Hough AJ Jr: Fibrin clot invasion by rabbit meniscal fibrochondrocytes in organ culture. *Trans Orthop Res Soc* 1987;12:470.

69. Thompson WO, Thaete FL, Fu FH, Dye SF: Tibial meniscal dynamics using three-dimensional reconstruction of magnetic resonance images. *Am J Sports Med* 1991;19:210–215.

70. Muller W (ed): *The Knee: Form, Function, and Ligament Reconstruction.* Berlin, Germany, Springer-Verlag, 1983.

71. Dowdy PA, Miniaci A, Arnoczky SP, Fowler PJ, Boughner DR: The effect of cast immobilization on meniscal healing: An experimental study in the dog. *Am J Sports Med* 1995;23:721–728.

72. Fitzgibbons RE, Shelbourne KD: "Aggressive" nontreatment of lateral meniscal tears seen during anterior cruciate ligament reconstruction. *Am J Sports Med* 1995;23:156–159.

73. Asik M, Sener N, Akpinar S, Durmaz H, Goksan A: Strength of different meniscus suturing techniques. *Knee Surg Sports Traumatol Arthrosc* 1997;5:80–83.

74. Rimmer MG, Nawana NS, Keene GC, Pearcy MJ: Failure strengths of different meniscal suturing techniques. *Arthroscopy* 1995;11:146–150.

75. Barrett GR, Richardson K, Ruff CG, Jones A: The effect of suture type on meniscus repair: A clinical analysis. *Am J Knee Surg* 1997;10:2–9.

76. Eggli S, Wegmuller H, Kosina J, Huckell C, Jakob RP: Long-term results of arthroscopic meniscal repair: An analysis of isolated tears. *Am J Sports Med* 1995;23:715–720.

77. Zhang Z, Arnold JA: Trephination and suturing of avascular meniscal tears: A clinical study of the trephination procedure. *Arthroscopy* 1996;12:726–731.

78. Zhang Z, Arnold JA, Williams T, McCann B: Repairs by trephination and suturing of longitudinal injuries in the avascular area of the meniscus in goats. *Am J Sports Med* 1995;23:35–41.

79. Fox JM, Rintz KG, Ferkel RD: Trephination of incomplete meniscal tears. *Arthroscopy* 1993;9:451–455.

80. Cannon WD Jr: Arthroscopic meniscal repair, in McGinty JB, Caspari RB, Jackson RW, Poehling GG (eds): *Operative Arthroscopy.* New York, NY, Raven Press, 1991, pp 237–251.

81. Cannon WD, Morgan CD: Meniscal repair: Part II. Arthroscopic repair techniques. *J Bone Joint Surg* 1994;76A:294–311.

82. Henning CE, Lynch MA, Yearout KM, Vequist SW, Stallbaumer RJ, Decker KA: Arthroscopic meniscal repair using an exogenous fibrin clot. *Clin Orthop* 1990;252:64–72.

83. Henning CE, Yearout KM, Vequist SW, Stallbaumer RJ, Decker KA: Use of the fascia sheath coverage and exogenous fibrin clot in the treatment of complex meniscal tears. *Am J Sports Med* 1991;19:626–631.

84. Barrett GR, Treacy SH: Use of the T-fix suture anchor in fascial sheath reconstruction of complex meniscal tears. *Arthroscopy* 1996;12:251–255.

85. Djurasovic M, Aldridge JW, Grumbles R, Rosenwasser MP, Howell D, Ratcliffe A: Knee joint immobilization decreases aggrecan gene expression in the meniscus. *Am J Sports Med* 1998;26:460–466.

86. Rosenberg TD, Paulos LE, Wnorowski DC, Gurley WD: Arthroscopic surgery: Meniscus refixation and meniscus healing. *Orthopade* 1990;19:82–89.

87. Brown GC, Rosenberg TD, Deffner KT: Inside-out meniscal repair using zone-specific instruments. *Am J Knee Surg* 1996;9:144–150.

88. Rosenberg TD, Scott SM, Coward DB, et al: Arthroscopic meniscal repair evaluated with repeat arthroscopy. *Arthroscopy* 1986;2:14–20.

89. Morgan CD, Wojtys EM, Casscells CD, Casscells SW: Arthroscopic meniscal repair evaluated by second-look arthroscopy. *Am J Sports Med* 1991;19:632–637.

90. DeHaven KE, Black KP, Griffiths HJ: Open meniscus repair: Technique and two to nine year results. *Am J Sports Med* 1989;17:788–795.

91. Cannon WD Jr, Vittori JM: The incidence of healing in arthroscopic meniscal repairs in anterior cruciate ligament-reconstructed knees versus stable knees. *Am J Sports Med* 1992;20:176–181.

92. Committee on Complications of the Arthroscopy Association of North America: Complications in arthroscopy: The knee and other joints. *Arthroscopy* 1986;2:253–258.

93. Austin KS, Sherman OH: Complications of arthroscopic meniscal repair. *Am J Sports Med* 1993;21:864–868.

94. Stone RG, Frewin PR, Gonzales S: Long-term assessment of arthroscopic meniscus repair: A two- to six-year follow-up study. *Arthroscopy* 1990;6:73–78.

95. Austin KS: Complications of arthroscopic meniscal repair. *Clin Sports Med* 1996;15:613–619.

96. Johnson LL: Meniscus repair: The outside-in technique, in Jackson DW (ed): *Master Techniques in Orthopaedic Surgery: Reconstructive Knee Surgery*. New York, NY, Raven Press, 1995, pp 51–68.

97. Rodeo SA, Warren RF: Meniscal repair using the outside-to-inside technique. *Clin Sports Med* 1996;15:469–481.

98. Johnson L: Meniscus repair: The outside-in technique, in Jackson DW (ed): *Master Techniques in Orthopaedic Surgery*. New York, NY, Raven Press, 1995, pp 51-68.

99. Rodeo SA, Warren RF, Arnoczky SP: Meniscal repair using an exogenous fibrin clot. *Tech Orthop* 1993;8:113–119.

100. Nicholas SJ, Rodeo SA, Ghelman B, et al: Arthroscopic meniscal repair using the outside-in technique. *Arthroscopy,* in press.

101. van Trommel MF, Simonian PT, Potter HG, Wickiewicz TL: Different regional healing rates with the outside-in technique for meniscal repair. *Am J Sports Med* 1998;26:446–452.

102. van Trommel MF, Potter HG, Ernberg LA, Simonian PT, Wickiewicz TL: The use of non-contrast magnetic resonance imaging in evaluating meniscal repair: Comparison with conventional arthrography. *Arthroscopy* 1998;14:2–8.

103. Morgan CD: The "all-inside" meniscus repair. *Arthroscopy* 1991;7:120-125.

104. Barrett GR, Richardson K, Koenig V: T-Fix endoscopic meniscal repair: Technique and approach to different types of tears. *Arthroscopy* 1995; 11:245–251.

105. Barrett GR, Treacy SH, Ruff CG: The T-Fix technique for endoscopic meniscus repair: Technique, complications, and preliminary results. *Am J Knee Surg* 1996;9:151–156.

106. Albrecht-Olsen P, Kristensen G, Tormala P: Meniscus bucket-handle fixation with an absorbable Biofix tack: Development of a new technique. *Knee Surg Sports Traumatol Arthrosc* 1993,1:104–106.

107. Albrecht-Olsen P, Lind T, Kristensen G, Falkenberg B: Failure strength of a new meniscus arrow repair technique: Biomechanical comparison with horizontal suture. *Arthroscopy* 1997;13:183–187.

108. Dervin GF, Downing KJ, Keene GC, McBride DG: Failure strengths of suture versus biodegradable arrow for meniscal repair: An in vitro study. *Arthroscopy* 1997;13:296–300.

109. Boenisch UW, Faber KJ, Ciarelli M, et al: Pull-out strength and stiffness of meniscus repair using absorbable arrows vs Ty-cron vertical and horizontal loop sutures. *Am J Sports Med,* in press.

110. Koukoubis TD, Glisson RR, Feagin JA Jr, et al: Meniscal fixation with an absorbable staple: An experimental study in dogs. *Knee Surg Sports Traumatol Arthrosc* 1997;5:22–30.

111. Kent RH, Pope CF, Lynch JK, Jokl P: Magnetic resonance imaging of the surgically repaired meniscus: Six-month follow-up. *Magn Reson Imaging* 1991;9:335–341.

112. Deutsch AL, Mink JH, Fox JM, et al: Peripheral meniscal tears: MR findings after conservative treatment or arthroscopic repair. *Radiology* 1990;176:485–488.

113. Ritchie JR, Miller MD, Bents RT, Smith DK: Meniscal repair in the goat model: The use of healing adjuncts on central tears and the role of magnetic resonance arthrography in repair evaluation. *Am J Sports Med* 1998;26:278–284.

114. Tenuta JJ, Arciero RA: Arthroscopic evaluation of meniscal repairs: Factors that effect healing. *Am J Sports Med* 1994:22:797–802.

115. Rubman MH, Noyes FR, Barber-Westin SD: Arthroscopic repair of meniscal tears that extend into the avascular zone: A review of 198 single and complex tears. *Am J Sports Med* 1998; 26:87–95.

116. Horibe S, Shino K, Maeda A, Nakamura N, Matsumoto N, Ochi T: Results of isolated meniscal repair evaluated by second-look arthroscopy. *Arthroscopy* 1996;12:150–155.

117. Barber FA, Click SD: Meniscus repair rehabilitation with concurrent anterior cruciate reconstruction. *Arthroscopy* 1997;13:433–437.

118. Jensen NC, Riis J, Robertsen K, Holm AR: Arthroscopic repair of the ruptured meniscus: One to 6.3 years follow up. *Arthroscopy* 1994;10:211–214.

119. Kimura M, Shirakura K, Hasegawa A, Kobuna Y, Niijima M: Second look arthroscopy after meniscal repair: Factors affecting the healing rate. *Clin Orthop* 1995;314:185–191.

120. Miller MD, Ritchie JR, Gomez BA, Royster RM, DeLee JC: Meniscal repair: An experimental study in the goat. *Am J Sports Med* 1995;23:124–128.

121. Port J, Jackson DW, Lee TQ, Simon TM: Meniscal repair supplemented with exogenous fibrin clot and autogenous cultured marrow cells in the goat model. *Am J Sports Med* 1996;24:547–555.

122. DeHaven KE, Lohrer WA, Lovelock JE: Long-term results of open meniscal repair. *Am J Sports Med* 1995;23:524–530.

123. Klein L, Heiple KG, Torzilli PA, Goldberg VM, Burstein AH: Prevention of ligament and meniscus atrophy by active joint motion in a non-weight-bearing model. *J Orthop Res* 1989;7:80–85.

124. Shelbourne KD, Johnson GE: Locked bucket-handle meniscal tears in knees with chronic anterior cruciate ligament deficiency. *Am J Sports Med* 1993;21:779–782.

125. Barber FA: Abstract: Unrestricted rehabilitation of meniscus repairs. *Arthroscopy* 1994;10:353.

126. Buseck MS, Noyes FR: Arthroscopic evaluation of meniscal repairs after anterior cruciate ligament reconstruction and immediate motion. *Am J Sports Med* 1991;19:489–494.

127. Shelbourne KD, Patel DV, Adsit WS, Porter DA: Rehabilitation after meniscal repair. *Clin Sports Med* 1996;15:595–612.

128. Ochi M, Mochizuki Y, Deie M, Ikuta Y: Augmented meniscal healing with free synovial autografts: An organ culture model. *Arch Orthop Trauma Surg* 1996;115:123–126.

129. Stone KR, Rodkey WG, Webber RJ, McKinney L, Steadman JR: Future directions: Collagen-based prostheses for meniscal regeneration. *Clin Orthop* 1990;252:129–135.

130. Stone KR, Steadman JR, Rodkey WG, Li ST: Regeneration of meniscal cartilage with use of a collagen scaffold: Analysis of preliminary data. *J Bone Joint Surg* 1997;79A:1770–1777.

131. Milachowski KA, Weismeier K, Wirth CJ, Kohn D: Abstract: Meniscus transplantation: Experimental study and first clinical report. *Am J Sports Med* 1987;15:626.

INDEX

Page numbers in bold italics refer to figures or figure legends.

A

Abrasion, synovial. *See* Synovial abrasion

All-inside repair
    complications, 44, 49
    techniques, 40–49

Allograft
    suturing, 35

Anatomy
    gross 2, 3
    meniscofemoral ligaments, 4
    vascular 6–7, *6–7*

Annandale, Thomas, 1, 7

Anterior cruciate ligament (ACL)
    reconstruction, 21
    tear, 11

Arrows. *See* Meniscus arrow repair

B

Biochemistry
    cell types, 4
    extracellular matrix, 4–5, 4

Blood supply
    menisci, 6–7, *6–8*
    role in healing, 7

Bucket handle tears, 20, 24, 43, 44

C

Cannula
    double lumen slotted, 33, *33*
    fibrin clot placement, *32*
    use, *27–28*, 30, *30, 33*

Collagen, 4

Complications
    all-inside repair, 44, 49
    Henning repair, 24
    inside-out repair, 33–34
    outside-in repair, 38

Compressive forces. *See* Weightbearing

D

Degenerative tears, 28

Double-barrel cannula technique, 12, *12*

E

Elastin, 4

Ethicon, *22*

Extracellular matrix, 4–5

F

Fibrin clot, 21, *27,* 37, 39, 51
    healing, 9, *10*
    placement, *23,* 31, *38*
    placement with cannula, *32*
    preparation, 22, *22*
    role in healing, 7

Fibrochondrocytes, 4
    and healing, **17**

Fingerstick injuries, avoiding, 18

Flap tears, 28

Function
    menisci, 5, 6

G

Genicular artery, 6

Glycoproteins, matrix. *See* Matrix glycoproteins

H

Healing
    amorphous debris buildup, **17**
    exogenous fibrin clot, 9
    fibrin clot, 7, 10, **10**
    fibrochondrocytes, **17**
    Henning repair, 25–27
    menisci, **7**, 7–10
    outside-in repair, 39–40
    results, **25**
    role of blood supply, 7
    synovial abrasion, 9, **10**
    T-fix suture anchor repair, 44
    vascular access channels, 9
    zone-specific repair, 32

Henning, Charles, 2, **2**, 14

Henning repair, 2
    complications, 24
    healing, 25–27
    instruments, 14, **15**
    rehabilitation, 24–25
    results, 25–27
    technique, 13–27

History
    meniscal repair, 1, 2

Horizontal cleavage tears, 11, 28

I

Ikeuchi, Hiroshi, 2, **2**

Indications
    meniscal repair, **11,** 11–12
    outside-in repair, 34–35
    zone-specific repair, 28

Inside-out repair
    complications, 33–34
    Henning repair, 13–27
    lateral meniscal repair, 22–24
    medial meniscus repair, 13–22
    technique, 13–34
    techniques, other, 32–33

J

Joint stability
    meniscal function, 5

K

Keith needles, 16, **17**

King, Don, 1, **1,** 7

Knee
    gross anatomy, 3
    joint stability, meniscal function, 5
    medial compartment, **3**
    medial compartment collapse, **5**
    proprioceptive structures, meniscal function, 6

Knee distractor
    use, **15**

Knee flexion
    menisci, 10

L

Lateral meniscal repair, 22–24, **23, 26, 30**

Ligament, anterior meniscofemoral, 4

Ligament of Humphrey.
    See Ligament, anterior meniscofemoral

Ligament of Wrisberg.
  See Ligament, posterior meniscofemoral

Ligament, posterior meniscofemoral, 4

Load transmission
  meniscal function, 5

M

Matrix glycoproteins, 4

McMurray test, 28

Medial collateral ligament (MCL) release, 21

Medial meniscus repair, 13–22, **26,** 30

Meniscus repair
  arthroscopic vs. open, 2
  complications of, 24, 33–34, 38, 44, 49
  discussion, 50–52
  future directions, 52–53
  history, 1-2
  indications, **11,** 11–12
  instruments, 15, **15**
  rehabilitation after, 24, 32, 38–39
  results, 25–27, **25–27,** 32, 39–40, 43–44
  techniques, 12–24, 27, 28–32, 35–38, 40–43,
    45–48

Meniscectomy
  arthritis, historical studies, 1
  medial compartment collapse, **5**
  partial, rationale, 8

Menisci
  biochemistry, 4–5
  blood supply, 6–7, **6–7,** 8–10, **8–10**
  cells, 4
  collagen fibers, 4, **4**
  elastin, 4
  fibrochondrocytes, 4
  function, 1, 5–6
  gross anatomy, 2, 3

healing, 1, **7,** 7–10
historical studies, 1
knee flexion, 10
lateral, anatomy, 3
matrix glycoproteins, 4
medial, anatomy, 3
medial, transection, **8**
motion, 10
proteoglycans, 4
segments, missing, 24
ultrastructure, 4
vascular anatomy, 6–7, **6–8**
weightbearing, 11

Meniscus arrow repair
  pullout strength, 44–45
  technique, 44–49

Meniscus arrows, 45
  instruments, **46**
  placement, **45-46, 48**
  preparation, **47**

Missing meniscal segments, 24

Motion
  menisci, 10

N

Needles 17, 42
  bending, 18, **18**
  Nitinol, 32, **33**
  placement, 37
  plastic covered, 42
  single, passage, 12, **12**
  spinal, **16, 35,** 42, **43**

Nerve injuries
  peroneal, 38
  Saphenous, 34, 38, 40

O

Oblique flap tears, 23, 24

Outside-in repair
    complications, 38
    healing, 39–40
    indications, 34–35
    rehabilitation, 38–39
    special technical considerations, 37–38
    technique, 34–40

P

Peripheral capsular detachment. *See* Red-red tear

Pins
    stabilizing, *46*

Posteromedial compartment
    inspection, *14*

Proprioceptive structures
    meniscal function, 6

Proteoglycans, 4

R

Rasping, 15–16

Red-red tear, 6, 8, 11

Red-white tear, 11, 28
    arthroscopic view, *9*
    healing, 8

Rehabilitation
    Henning repair, 24–25, 52
    outside-in repair, 38–39
    zone-specific repair, 32

S

Shock absorption
    meniscal function, 5

Single-needle passage, 12, *12*

Spinal needle
    placement, *43*
    use, *16*, *35*, 42

Staples, *49*
    use, 49

Suture anchor
    placement, *43*

Suture hook
    instruments, *41*

Suture hook repair
    technique, 40–41

Sutures
    absorbable, 30
    Ethibond, *22*
    knots, *42*
    mattress, *36*, *44*
    nonabsorbable, 30
    organization, *21*
    orientation, 12, *12*
    placement, 17–19, *17–21*, 23, *24*, 30–31, *30–31*, *34–36*, *38*, *41*
    retrieval, *41*
    stacking, *20*
    T-fix, *42*

Synovial abrasion, *16*
    healing, 9, *10*

T

T-fix suture anchor repair
    healing, 44
    technique, 41–44

Tacks, *49*

Tears
    blood supply, 8–10, *9*
    broken bucket-handle, 24
    degenerative, 28
    displaced bucket-handle, 20
    flap, 28

horizontal cleavage, 28
oblique flap, 24
radial split, 11, 23, 24

Techniques
all-inside repair, 40–49
double-barrel cannula, 12, *12*
general, 12
Henning repair, 13–27
inside-out repair, 13–34
inside-out repair, other, 32–33
lateral meniscal repair, 22–24, *23*
medial meniscus repair, 13–22
meniscus arrow repair, 44–49
outside-in repair, 34–40
single-needle passage, 12, *12*
suture hook repair, 40–41
T-fix suture anchor repair, 41–44
zone-specific repair, 27–32

Thigh holder
use, *13*

Tibial plateau, *3*

U

Ultrastructure
menisci, 4

V

Vasculature
access channels, 9
peripheral, 9

W

Weightbearing, 11, 38

White-white tear, 9, 10, 31
fibrin clot, *9*
healing, 8

Z

Zone-specific repair
healing, 32
indications, 28
rehabilitation, 32
technique, 27–32